TRAIN LIKE A
BODYBUILDER
AT HOME

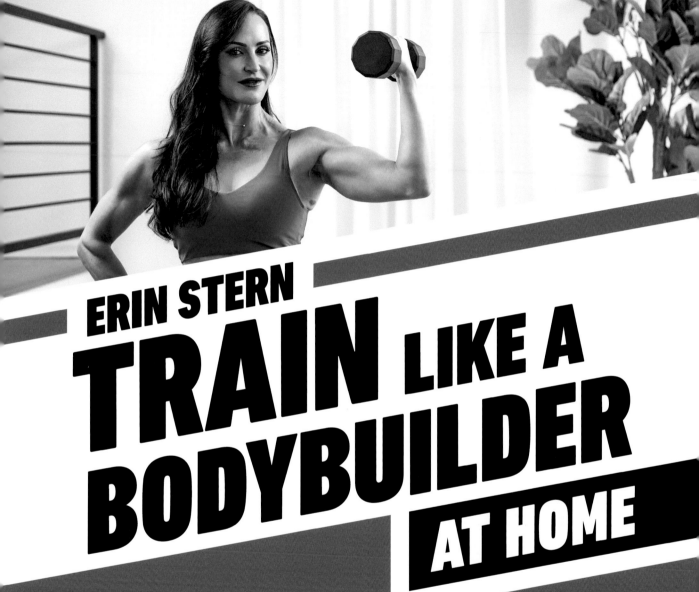

ERIN STERN
TRAIN LIKE A BODYBUILDER
AT HOME

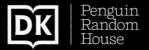

Publisher Mike Sanders
Senior Editor Brook Farling
Art & Design Director William Thomas
Compositor Ayanna Lacey
Photographer Kelley Jordan Schuyler
Proofreader Lisa Starnes
Indexer Jessica Crooks

First American Edition, 2022
Published in the United States by DK Publishing
6081 E. 82nd Street, Indianapolis, Indiana 46250
Copyright © 2022 Erin Stern
22 23 24 25   10 9 8 7 6 5 4 3 2 1
001-323164-NOV2022

Library of Congress Catalog Number: 2022934282
ISBN: 978-0-7440-3490-5

DK books are available at special discounts when purchased in bulk for sales promotions, premiums, fundraising, or educational use. For details, contact: SpecialSales@dk.com

Printed and bound in China

for the curious
www.dk.com

CONTENTS

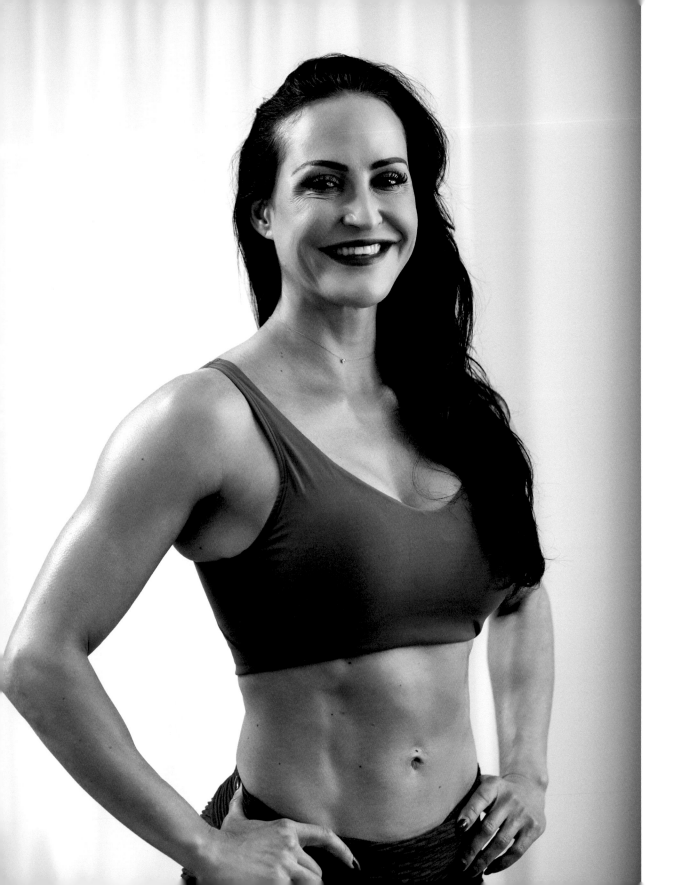

ABOUT THE AUTHOR

From a young age, Erin Stern has loved fitness. She grew up riding horses and later started running track, eventually earning athletic and academic scholarships to attend the University of Florida, where she competed in the high jump, pentathlon, and heptathlon. She was a Junior All-American in the high jump and earned All-SEC academic honors each year she attended college.

After college, Erin jumped 5 feet 11 inches (1.80 meters), just missing the Olympic qualifying standard for the high jump by 3 centimeters. It was this disappointment that sparked her love of bodybuilding. After four weeks of prep, she stepped onto a stage at a small local show and won the overall figure title. Two months later, she stood on stage at the NPC Nationals as the overall Figure Champion and a new IFBB Figure Pro. During her figure career, Erin won 11 IFBB Pro League titles, including the Figure Olympia twice. She left bodybuilding in 2014, but she missed it so much that she went back to compete again, this time in the bikini division. In 2019, Erin traveled to Vietnam for the Vietnam Muscle Contest and won her Pro card in IFBB Bikini. Since then, she has achieved several top-five finishes, a Pro victory, and a top-15 placing at the 2021 Bikini Olympia.

Erin continues to compete, but her focus is coaching others to get into the best shapes of their lives and to help them sustain their fitness. She's helped thousands of people accomplish this goal. She combines her track-and-field training with bodybuilding hypertrophy training to create interesting, fun, challenging, and effective training programs for people of all ages.

ACKNOWLEDGMENTS

Thank you to everyone at DK Books for making this book possible. Special thanks to Brook for his excellent attention to detail and for editing and perfecting every page in this book. Thank you to Becky for giving this book flow, structure, and layouts that are not only easy to follow but lovely to look at. Thank you to William for his keen design eye, organizational skills, and creative guidance. Thank you to Mike for this tremendous opportunity and for enriching people's lives with books.

Thank you to my parents, Gail and Ira, for telling me that I could accomplish anything I set my mind and heart to. Thank you for involving me in athletics and teaching me to be a strong girl. You gave me the confidence to pursue my dreams and to ultimately achieve them.

Thank you to my fiancé, Evan, for being my best friend, for being so supportive, and for being a part of this book.

Thank you to my favorites in the fitness industry: Dr. Brad Schoenfeld, Dr. Mike Israetel, Andrew Huberman, Nick Tumminello, Dr. Rhonda Patrick, and Dr. Gabrielle Lyon. You have paved the way for the combination of science, healthy living, and smart training.

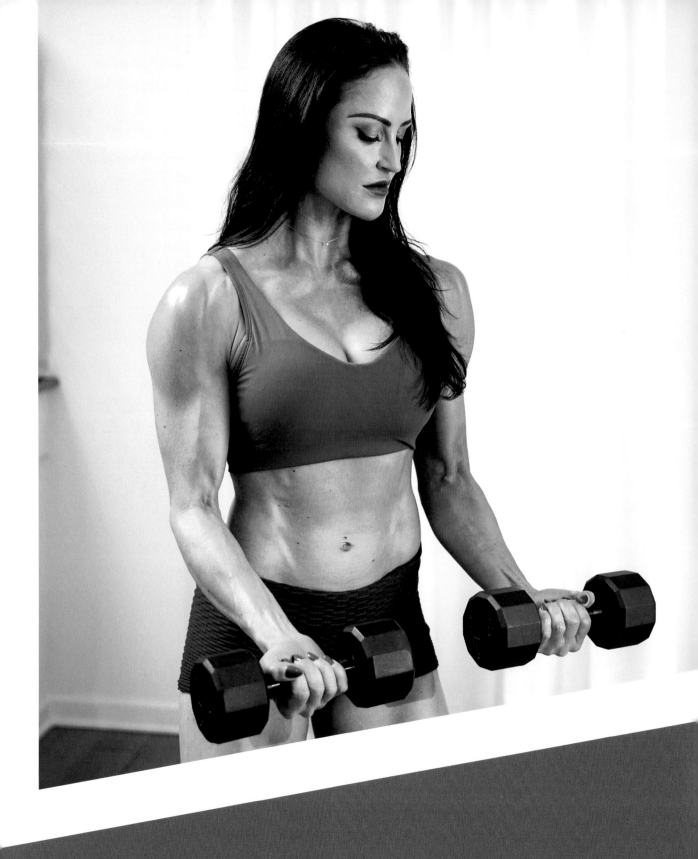

INTRODUCTION

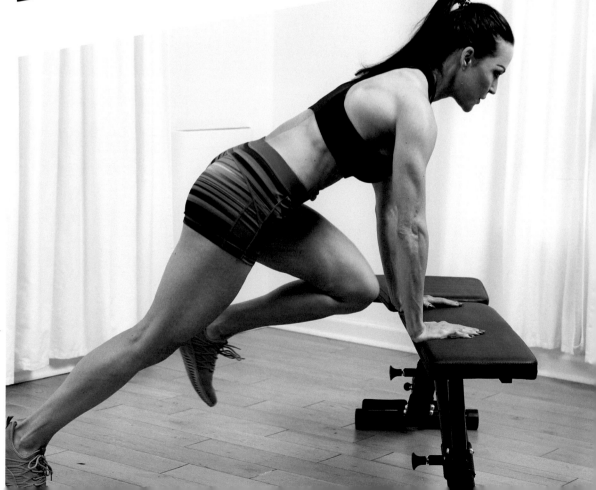

WHY TRAIN LIKE A BODYBUILDER AT HOME?

When most people think of bodybuilding, they probably think of bodybuilding competitions and people with well-developed muscles carrying big jugs of water as they work their way around the gym. These things are a part of bodybuilding—albeit the extreme part—but if you've ever lifted weights with the intent of shaping or changing your physique, you are a bodybuilder, too! Bodybuilding is not about haphazardly throwing weights around a gym; it's about putting forth a focused effort to build strategic muscle to create a physique. Bodybuilding also can be one of the most rewarding pastimes you'll ever partake in.

CONVENIENCE

One of the most common questions about bodybuilding is if you have to go to a gym to do it, and the answer is no! A lot of people don't want to train in a gym because they think they have to push heavy weights and use complex machines to get the same muscle a bodybuilder gets in a gym, but that's simply not true. You can train like a bodybuilder almost anywhere. You can mimic almost any exercise at home that you would perform in a gym, and you don't need heavy weights to do it. You just need some basic equipment, a well-defined training plan, and the commitment to stick to your workouts. You don't have to pay for a gym membership, you don't have to fight crowds, and you don't have to wipe down equipment. If you want to build your ideal physique but you don't want to go to a gym to do it, you can still get serious results while training at home.

AESTHETIC BENEFITS

The secret to creating epic proportions is training the same way a bodybuilder trains. To create a smaller waist, a bodybuilder builds upper-body muscle to create an impressive *V-taper,* which is the distinct look a bodybuilder gets by building broad upper-body musculature. Bodybuilders also want strong curves, and they achieve this by training their delts, upper back, glutes, and legs. These are the primary strategies bodybuilders employ to build amazing musculature. You'll also notice your clothing fits better and your skin appears tighter and glowing. And even if you're just looking to improve muscle definition, bodybuilding will help you build visible muscle while improving your overall definition. And as a bonus, you get to wear the results of your hard work wherever you go! Whenever you walk into a room, your hard work, dedication, and discipline will be recognized.

PHYSICAL BENEFITS

Training like a bodybuilder reduces your chances of injury. Most people are born with a dominant side. And through everyday life and athletic activites, that stronger, dominant side can become even more developed. This can lead to asymmetries. Bodybuilding evens out asymmetries and "brings up" your nondominant arm or leg to create a more uniform appearance while improving strength and reducing the chance of injury. Not only does bodybuilding give you the opportunity to create your ideal physique, it also is a stress reliever, a metabolism booster, and the closest thing science has found to being a fountain of youth.

As you train, you may notice a change in your posture as bodybuilding not only adds muscle to your frame but also improves flexibility through stretching as you go through a full range of motion on your lifts. Improved posture leads to improved self-confidence. This can boost your sense of well-being and decrease stress levels.

Building muscle enhances your metabolism and can improve insulin sensitivity. This becomes especially important as you age as the body usually becomes more insulin resistant and more likely to develop type 2 diabetes or mitochondrial dysfunction. After the age of 30, people can lose as much as 3–5 percent of their muscle mass per decade. This loss can contribute to lower hormone levels, weakness, and lower quality of life. Bodybuilding prevents *sarcopenia,* which is the accelerated loss of muscle mass and muscle function, and can actually reverse it. As you build muscle, your body composition changes, too. Losing fat becomes easier, and while you may find that your weight changes drastically, your clothes will fit better and you may not have to focus as much on dieting to maintain your weight. Muscle protects your joints and builds bone density. You'll enjoy better balance, less risk of injury, and stronger bones. This means a higher quality of life and a longer lifespan.

We often think about lifespan and wanting to live a long life, but it's not as much about the years as it is about the quality of life and being in good health to enjoy it. So when you think about bodybuilding and bodybuilders, don't just think about creating your ideal physique and building your body, think about how much it's going to improve your life! Now, let's work together to get stronger, better, and healthier!

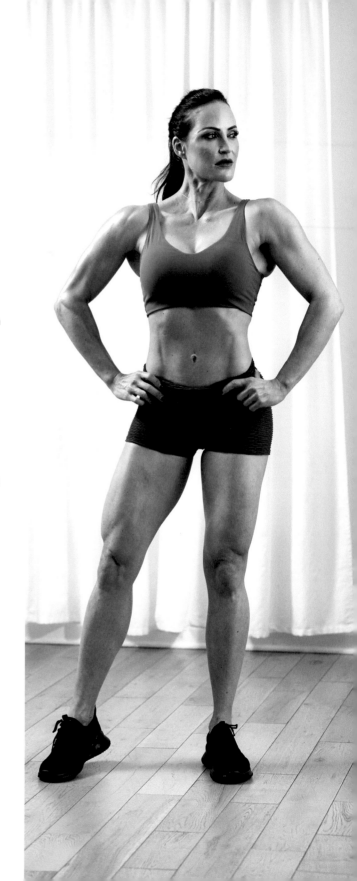

THE SIX FUNDAMENTAL COMPOUND MOVEMENTS

The foundations of most strength-training workouts should be comprised of six basic types of movement: squat, hip hinge, vertical press, vertical pull, horizontal press, and horizontal pull. These basic movements are known as *compound lifts* or *multi-joint movements,* meaning multiple muscles are trained by the movement. *Isolation movements* have a place in your workouts and will add shape to individual muscles, but they tend to only target individual muscles and are used to sculpt, shape, and "bring up" certain areas of a muscle. Compound movements create maximum calorie burn. A good example of a compound movement is a push-up, which will train the chest, core, front delts, and triceps. By emphasizing these six fundamental compound movements and their variations in your workouts, you'll be able to burn more calories and also train your muscles more effectively. This will help reduce the time you spend training and also help you see results more quickly. And you'll be able to create hundreds of variations from each basic movement, potentially giving you almost unlimited training options!

INCORPORATING ROTATIONAL WORK INTO YOUR ROUTINE

While not one of the six fundamental types of compound movement covered in this book, rotational exercises can help build core stability and strength, thus reducing injury risk. Rotational work is twisting in a transverse plane: picture throwing a baseball or swinging a golf club. When lifting weights, we're pulling or pushing with a tight core and only moving along one plane of motion. While this translates to increases in muscle mass, strength, speed, and power, it doesn't always translate to how we move in everyday life. Therefore, it's a good idea to add some rotational exercises and rotational lunges to your routine.

SQUAT

Often called the "king of exercises," the squat targets almost every muscle in the legs and glutes. It also strengthens the core and improves overall balance and stability. You may consider the squat a lower-body exercise, but with home-friendly 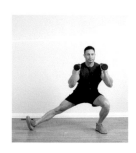 variations, you'll often also be engaging your back, shoulders, and arms. The most well-known variation of the squat is the barbell back squat, which is popular among powerlifters and gymgoers. It's a difficult movement to master, however, and many home gyms aren't equipped with squat racks, so in this book you'll find exercises like the goblet squat, Spanish squat, and Cossack squat, along with split squats and single-leg squats, that can all be effective and challenging variations of the barbell back squat.

HIP HINGE

Many hip hinge movements target the posterior chain, which includes the hamstrings, glutes, and lower back. Not only do hip hinge movements add muscle, they can greatly improve power and speed, which translates well to other lifts and to daily 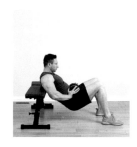 movements, such as bending over to pick things up or lifting heavy objects. Strengthening your lower back can reduce lower-back pain, too. At first glance, the squat and hip hinge can look similar, but there's a simple way to tell them apart: the squat is a knee-dominant lift, whereas the hip hinge is a hip-dominant lift. Some examples of hip hinge exercises you'll find in this book include dumbbell deadlifts, hip thrusts, good mornings, and dumbbell swings.

VERTICAL PRESS

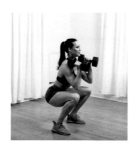

One vertical pressing movement can simultaneously and effectively target the shoulders, chest, triceps, upper back, and core. If you're looking to build capped shoulders and tie upper-body musculature together aesthetically, vertical press movements should be staples in your training routines. Choosing to do these movements while standing will engage the core muscles more effectively and provide more difficult variations, which is particularly important if you have a limited amount of weight in your home gym. Some examples of vertical press exercises that you find in this book include shoulder press, Y-press, pike press, dips, and thrusters.

HORIZONTAL PRESS

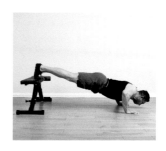

Horizontal pressing movements involve flexion and extension of the elbows in a horizontal line away from your body. Horizontal pressing movements target the upper body, including the chest, front delts, triceps, and core. These movements can help create width in your body from front to back, which can balance the upper and lower body and create the illusion of a smaller waist. Keep in mind that the extension doesn't have to be precisely horizontal as you can perform movements on a decline or on an incline. Some examples of horizontal pressing exercises include flat, incline, and decline bench press; push-ups; and decline push-ups.

VERTICAL PULL

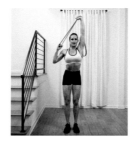

Vertical pulling exercises complement vertical pressing exercises perfectly. While the chest and triceps will work to stabilize the body during vertical pulls, it's the back and biceps that are the major weight movers during this type of movement. Additionally, smaller back muscles like teres and rhomboids are also trained. Wider-grip vertical pulling exercises work to really bring out the V-taper while more narrow-grip variations can hit the mid-back and chest. The most common vertical pulling exercise is a pull-up, but other examples that you'll find in this book include pull-downs, upright rows, and shrugs.

HORIZONTAL PULL

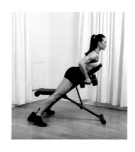

Horizontal pulling involves the extension and flexion (or pulling toward you) of the elbows. This movement builds lats, biceps, rear delts, and many of the smaller muscles in the mid-back. Along with vertical pulling movements, horizontal pulling movements can improve your V-taper and balance your physique from upper body to lower body, particularly if you have dominant legs. Horizontal pulling can improve your deadlift and squat strength along with improving your posture. Horizontal pulling movements also tend to be kinder on shoulders than vertical pulling movements, and there are more at-home horizontal pulling options than vertical pulling options. Some examples of horizontal pulling exercises include dumbbell rows, cable rows, supine rows, low rows, and bent over rows.

BASIC STRENGTH TRAINING PRINCIPLES

The same basic training concepts that apply to gym training still apply to home training. Techniques like supersets, giant sets, and circuits can all be used at home to save time and increase calorie burn. And principles like frequency, volume, training close to failure, tempo and tension, partial reps, and isometric holds can all still be utilized effectively, though they may need to be adjusted slightly for training at home since home equipment is limited. Here are the basic strength training principles that every bodybuilder needs to know.

FREQUENCY

When it comes to gaining or maintaining muscle, it's important to train target muscles often. A few factors must be taken into consideration when planning exercise frequency. First, you should decide how many days per week you can train. Be realistic when doing so; it's better to underestimate the number of days per week you can train rather than overestimate and miss workouts. It's also important to program in recovery time between training sessions. This recovery time is necessary for resting muscle groups as well as tendons, joints, and the central nervous system. If your workouts are short and lower in volume, you can potentially train each muscle group more frequently. If your workouts are longer and higher in volume, however, you may need more time to recover before the next session. A good range for training is 4 to 6 days per week as this will allow you the most flexibility in programming effective workouts, yet also give you enough time to recover well and also make progress.

VOLUME

Training volume refers to the overall sets and reps you perform during individual workouts as well as for the entire week of training. It's best to start with the least amount of volume needed to produce changes in your physique and then slowly add volume each week. This will result in better progress, it will save you time, and it can help you avoid overreaching. Overreaching occurs when you habitually train muscle groups before they have recovered properly. This can cause injury and hinder progress. A good rule of thumb is to increase your volume by about 10 percent each week. As your muscles adapt and gain strength, you'll need to continue to challenge them to see results. This increase in volume is known as *progressive overload,* and it helps ensure gains in strength and size over time. Other ways to ensure progressive overload are lifting heavier weights each week and increasing exercise frequency. Since weight equipment tends to be limited at home, increasing volume over time is a great option for making gains.

TRAINING CLOSE TO FAILURE

Training to failure or close to failure can be an effective technique for home training. Since at-home training equipment is limited, increasing reps becomes necessary to continue adding muscle. Recent studies have shown that muscle gain occurs in all reps ranging from 5 to 30 reps, as long as at least 30 percent of your one-rep max is used. This means that you can make tremendous gains with much less weight than previously thought. But it's very important that each set be performed close to failure. A good rule of thumb for most exercises is to leave 1 to 4 reps "in the tank," meaning that you work a set until you feel you can only achieve 1 to 4 more reps in the set. This strategy can create enough stimulus to affect change in the muscles but without taxing your central nervous system. Sometimes it can still be effective to train to failure, also known as "AMRAP" or *as many reps as possible.* AMRAP sets are typically best done with bodyweight exercises or isolation exercises, with the goal of taxing your muscles but not frying yourself to the point where you can't train the next day.

TEMPO AND TENSION

Tempo is a key tool for any lifter who is looking to gain or maintain muscle, but it's even more important when it comes to training at home. You can increase exercise difficulty greatly by slowing down your lifting tempo. This increases the amount of tension and the duration of tension on the muscle, which can lead to increases in muscle size and strength. Another benefit of slowing the tempo of your lifting is improving mind-muscle connection. By slowing your tempo, you'll be able to perform stronger contractions of the muscles, which means you will not need as much volume to get the same results. When slowing down the tempo, it's usually best to focus on the negative, or *eccentric,* portion of the rep. Muscles are around 30 percent stronger during the negative portion of the rep compared to the *concentric* portion of the rep since most muscle damage occurs during the negative portion of the rep. This damage is actually a good thing as it forces the muscle to repair itself to be stronger and larger than it was before! Tension may also be added with the use of bands. Bands increase difficulty and allow you to add tension in ways that free weights can't. The result is a novel stimulus to the muscles, which can help cause muscle growth. Adding a band to lighter weights increases exercise difficulty dramatically, and it's also a great option for when you'd like to go heavier on an exercise but don't have a heavier set of dumbbells.

PARTIAL REPS

Another way to increase difficulty in home training is to add partial reps to a set. A partial rep is where you find the toughest portion within the range of motion of a rep and perform the reps strictly within that range. When it comes to training, the body can become accustomed to exercises—this can happen with the range of motion and angles or with frequently performed exercise variations. By shortening the range of motion, muscles are forced to adapt. An ideal approach is to add partial reps as part of your last set of an exercise. Partial reps can also be added as finishers or burnouts, which both can increase blood flow to the muscle.

ISOMETRIC HOLDS

Isometric holds are another way to increase tension within a muscle. An isometric hold is where you pause briefly during a rep, typically at the point of maximum muscle contraction. For example, when doing lateral raises, adding a 1- to 2-second pause at the mid-rep point will light up your delts and also improve mind-muscle connection. The brief pause can also allow you time to reset and ensure you're targeting the muscles you are working. Short isometric holds are also referred to as "pause" reps. Isometric holds can also be used for longer durations. They can help with fat burning, and when used with bodyweight exercises, they can improve strength without adding size. Long isometric holds also make good finishers and tough ab workouts. (If you have performed a wall sit or a plank, you have performed a long isometric hold.)

GRIP STYLES

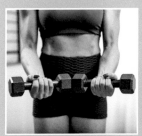

OVERHAND (PRONATED)

Grasp the weights with your palms facing down. (A *false grip* is an overhand grip without a thumb wrap.) Some lifters prefer to use a false grip, but it can be dangerous, so you should always wrap your thumbs around the bar.

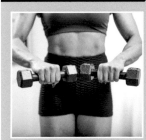

UNDERHAND (SUPINATED)

Grasp the weights with your palms facing upward. Underhand grips are most commonly used for pulling exercises and are particularly effective for training the biceps and the muscles in the front areas of the shoulders.

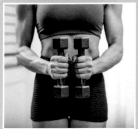

NEUTRAL

Grasp the weights with your palms facing each other. This position can help take stress off of the wrists, forearms, and shoulders. You can use a neutral grip when training with free weights or on machines, but not with a bar.

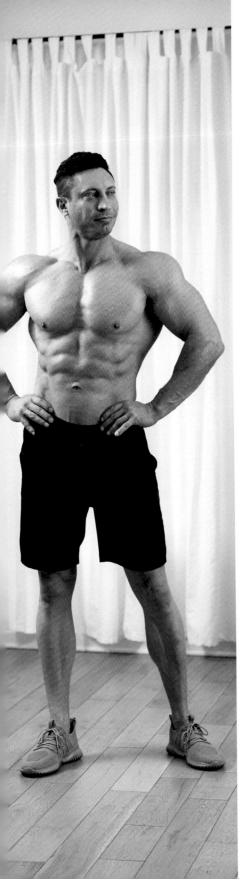

THE BASICS OF BUILDING MUSCLE

Adding muscle requires more than just performing daily workouts. You need to understand basic physiological principles of building muscle and basic training principles, as well as the essentials of proper nutrition that will give you the fuel you'll need for workouts, recovery, and muscle building. This all may seem like a lot to take in, but it's the basic knowledge you'll need to build your dream physique at home.

THE THREE PHYSIOLOGICAL PRINCIPLES OF MUSCLE GAIN

For maximum muscle gain, you need to increase three things: mechanical tension, metabolic stress, and muscle damage. If you can integrate even one of the following training principles into your training routine, you'll see results. And if you can incorporate all three into your routine, you'll leave no gains on the table.

MECHANICAL TENSION

Mechanical tension occurs when you lift heavy weights. This can be a challenge at home, but it can be done with bands and big compound movements, and by sticking to lower reps in the 5- to 10-rep range. Incorporating challenging bodyweight movements like pike push-ups can also help increase mechanical tension.

METABOLIC STRESS

Metabolic stress occurs when you're lifting light to moderate weight for high reps. (This is also known as "the pump.") This principle is excellent for at-home training, especially if you have limited equipment. Be sure that your sets are always about 1 to 4 reps from failure to help with muscle growth. When you employ this principle, your muscles will grow, but you won't necessarily gain strength.

MUSCLE DAMAGE

Muscle damage, though it sounds like something to avoid, is actually necessary for gaining muscle. The difference between this calculated microdamage and actual injury is that you are causing this controlled damage, or micro-tears, to the muscle fibers whenever you train. As the fibers heal, they will grow back even stronger and larger than before. Slowing down your tempo and also focusing on the negative, or eccentric portion of the rep are both effective ways to activate protein synthesis and repair microdamage in muscle fibers. This is great news when you're training at home as you can still see great results by performing your reps more slowly while using lighter weights.

THE BASIC TRAINING PRINCIPLES FOR GAINING MUSCLE

In addition to understanding how muscle is built, it's important to understand some basic training principles and how to apply them. By understanding these principles, you'll be able to determine how often you need to train, how many sets you need to do, and how often you should change things up.

VOLUME

Maximizing muscle growth requires hitting each muscle group with a certain amount of volume in sets and reps per week. Depending on your fitness level, recovery, and goals, that volume is typically between 10 to 20 sets per week. You can do one high-volume workout per week that satisfies the volume requirement, but the quality of the volume matters, too, so it can be beneficial to split up your training into two or three different sessions per week.

FREQUENCY

Each time you train a muscle, you increase muscle protein synthesis in that muscle, which creates more opportunity for growth. To make gains, you'll want to train each muscle group at least once per week; anything less than that and you could lose most of the adaptations you've created from previous workouts. Total body, high-frequency training splits often include exercises for the same muscle groups every day, but since the overall daily volume is low, you'll still be able to train with intensity and recover well. A typical bodybuilder "bro" split hits just one muscle group per day, with a lot of volume.

PROGRESSION

As you continue in a training program, you must include progression by continuing to challenge your muscles each week by either increasing the weight lifted or by increasing the volume. You can do both, but for home training it's more beneficial to increase volume. For example, if you're doing 3 sets of 8 reps during any given week, you may move to 3 sets of 9 reps the next week. A good rule of thumb is to shoot for a 10 percent increase in volume per week while following a program.

PRIORITIZATION

If you want to build capped delts or round glutes, prioritizing both of those muscle groups in your training splits with targeted exercise choices is important. For example, if your main goal is to build your shoulders, they should be targeted on day one of your workout split. And the first few exercises of that workout will be the ones that will best get you to your goal.

PATIENCE

Progress can be seen in just a few weeks when you're leaning down, but if your goal is muscle gain, it will take patience. Though you will see results in your first month of training, building lasting muscle mass takes at least 90 days. Someone new to lifting may add 1 to 2 pounds of muscle mass per month, but a seasoned lifter can expect to gain less. Don't fret if you're not experiencing the gains you want and as quickly as you might prefer—by focusing on adding strategic muscle, your results will still be impressive in due time.

NUTRITION

To build muscle as quickly as possible, you should focus on eating a slight surplus of calories each day. The surplus should be comprised of carbs and protein as both help with the muscle gain process. Overeating fats will cause you to gain fat more easily. If your goal is to gain muscle while losing fat, you can eat at maintenance calories to accomplish this. For most physique goals, a higher protein diet will help with muscle building, maintenance, recovery, and metabolism. (See the spreads on nutrition for detailed information on how to figure out your caloric needs and how to choose a nutrition plan.)

BUILDING MIND-MUSCLE CONNECTION

When you're training for muscle growth, you might hear the term "mind-muscle connection." If you're new to lifting or if you've never thought about focusing your mind specifically on a muscle while you're training, connecting your mind with a muscle might seem a little bit out there. But mind-muscle connection is an important component of effective training—it gives you the ability to isolate a muscle and perform stronger contractions with that specific muscle. By developing strong mind-muscle connection, you'll need less volume to see results than you normally would because you'll be less likely to work other unintended muscles. You'll also experience greater strength gains, better body awareness, and faster progress. When you're training at home, you may have limited equipment, so the ability to create strong mind-muscle connection will help make your workouts much more effective. Let's delve into how you can develop mind-muscle connection and the ways you can improve it.

START WITH
THE MUSCLES YOU CAN SEE

It's often easiest to start practicing mind-muscle connection with "mirror muscles," or the muscles you can see when you look in the mirror. These muscles include front delts, chest, biceps, abs, and quads. Single-arm or single-leg exercises can further help you focus on how a specific muscle moves and contracts. Watch your biceps as you do curls, and then close your eyes and try to *feel* the muscle working. Glance back at your biceps to reinforce both what you're seeing and feeling. If you have a floor-length mirror in your home gym, even better—you'll really be able to see the muscles work through a range of motion. Focus most on the middle portion of the rep, where the contraction is the strongest. Also focus on the eccentric portion of the rep, rather than the concentric portion of the rep.

TRAINING MUSCLES
YOU CAN'T SEE

When it comes to training muscles you can't see, you must rely on feel. The back, glutes, hamstrings, and rear delts can be tough to target without practice. Perfect your mind-muscle connection on the muscles you can see, and then move to the muscles you can't see. Go slowly, work with light weights or bands, and focus on the squeeze. If you have a lightweight floor mirror, bring it into your bathroom and position it on the floor and across from your bathroom mirror at an angle so you can see your lats, back, rear delts, and other muscles in one of the mirrors. Slowly extend your arms overhead, and pretend you're doing a lat pulldown. Next, pretend to perform a row. Get a good squeeze for each rep you perform, and watch your back in the mirror, then close your eyes and feel the squeeze. Open your eyes again and check the mirror for visual confirmation.

LIGHTEN UP,
SLOW DOWN, AND REPEAT

Because it takes concentrated effort to improve mind-muscle connection, it can help to use a lighter weight or a lighter resistance band when you're just starting to develop this skill. If you're lifting heavy, your focus can shift to just moving the weight and not moving the weight with certain muscles, which is more important. Slow down each rep. This will give you time to process the feeling, the contraction, and the movement itself. Once you begin to feel specific muscles firing, keep performing reps. Repetition improves retention. When you're done training and are at rest, your brain will process this new information and you'll become better at it with each session.

BE MINDFUL AND
LIFT WITH INTENTION

Another factor that can improve mind-muscle connection is lifting with intention and mindfulness. Visualize your muscles firing before an exercise, and keep your attention focused on the muscle you're working. Discipline yourself to stay focused on the muscle, especially during those last 2 to 3 reps when you might want to quit—those last few tough reps are where almost all gains are made. Know that all is not lost if you aren't able to stay focused or if you lose mind-muscle connection as you get tired or as your muscles fatigue. It can be normal to lose mind-muscle connection toward the end of a workout. Just keep pushing through. Consistency in training is key!

UNDERSTANDING MACRONUTRIENTS

While training is important for eliciting changes in your physique, proper nutrition is what makes those changes possible. Nutrition dictates if you'll gain muscle or lean down and how well you'll recover from previous training sessions. And while caloric intake is the driving factor behind weight gain or weight loss, macronutrients—or *macros* for short—are what matter for creating body composition. When it comes to daily meal planning, there are three macros to consider: protein, carbohydrates, and fats.

PROTEIN

Protein is the building block of every cell in the body. It aids recovery and helps with muscle building, it increases feelings of satiety, it boosts metabolism, and it has a mild diuretic effect. It's very important to note that the body cannot store protein, so it's important to eat protein at every meal and snack. A good goal is to aim for eating 1 gram of protein per 1 pound of weight. If your goal is fat loss, you can set your protein intake to 1 gram per pound of your estimated ideal body weight. If your goal is muscle gain, you can drop protein intake slightly to around 0.8 grams per 1 pound of body weight to allow for a higher carbohydrate intake, which can help with building muscle. Good sources of protein include lean meats, eggs, egg whites, seafood, low-fat dairy (like cottage cheese and Greek yogurt), and protein supplements. Vegan options include tempeh, seitan, tofu, and lean meat substitutes. Protein has a nutritional value of 4 calories per gram.

CARBOHYDRATES

Carbohydrates, or *carbs* for short, are the body's preferred energy source. Carbs are classified as either simple or complex. Simple carbs are made up of shorter chains of molecules and are much easier and quicker to digest. Simple carbs can be found in natural foods like fruits and milk, and in processed foods like table sugar and soft drinks. Complex carbs are comprised of longer chains of molecules, which are slower to digest and offer more sustained energy. Complex carbs also often contain higher amounts of fiber than simple carbs, which can help with satiety.

Carbs play a big role in building muscle as they aid not only in increased energy but also in recovery. Carbs are also known as *protein sparing,* which means they provide glucose for energy, which helps prevent the body from breaking down muscle for glucose. While eating protein at each meal and snack is recommended, you should think about eating most of your carbs when you're active. Carbs can be thought of as fuel, so you can "gas up" when you need energy or when you want to improve recovery. It can also be helpful to vary your carb sources both before and after working out. Before a workout, a meal with complex carbs and protein can give you sustained energy for the workout. After a workout, eating a meal comprised of protein and simple carbs or easy-to-digest complex carbs like white rice can be a good choice. Eating faster-digesting carbs means that your body will assimilate the meal more quickly and you'll also get a good head start on replenishing energy stores and recovery. Complex carb choices include all whole grains, oats, rice, beans, potatoes, and winter and summer squash. Simple carbs include fruits, fruit juices, processed foods, and syrups. Carbs have a nutritional value of 4 calories per gram.

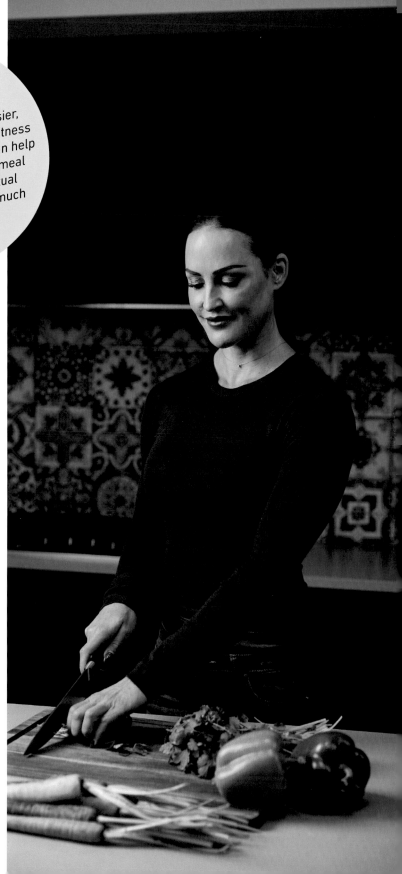

////////// **TIP** //////////
To make calculating and counting macronutrients easier, check out free apps like My Fitness Pal or Chronometer. These can help take the guesswork out of meal planning, making the actual planning and tracking a much easier process.

FATS ///

Unlike carbs, fats are essential for proper body function. The body can't make essential fatty acids on its own, so they must be consumed as part of a healthy diet. Fats necessitate cellular function, are involved in hormone production, protect your organs, carry fat-soluble vitamins, and offer a source of energy. The types of dietary fats you consume matter, so it's important to make good choices. Healthy fats include nuts, seeds, egg yolks, cold water fatty fish, avocados, and some oils like avocado or olive oil. The types of fats to avoid or at least limit include industrial seed and vegetable oils. They are high in omega-6 fatty acids, which can increase inflammation in the body which can lead to damage in the organs and joints over time as well as an increased risk of chronic disease. As a general guideline, try to consume fats when you're more sedentary, and try to limit your fat intake in your pre- and post-workout meals to 5 grams or less. Fats have over twice the caloric value of protein or carbs with 9 calories per gram.

DETERMINING CALORIC NEEDS

The human body and the way it functions is science, but there's also an art to it. No metabolism is the same; we burn more calories one day than we do the next. Therefore, it's very important to track your caloric intake, at least when you're first starting out with your training. This will give you the information you need to adjust your caloric intake as your body changes. (Using a free app like My Fitness Pal can make tracking much easier.)

The first step to figuring out caloric needs is to determine your basal metabolic rate, or BMR. This is the amount of energy or calories you need just to keep your body alive. Never allow your caloric intake to drop below your BMR. By staying at or above your BMR, you'll help prevent your body from hitting a plateau and slowing down your metabolism. There are several calculators online that will help you determine your BMR (Active.com has one that I like to use.)

Once you have calculated your BMR, the next step is to estimate your caloric needs based on your training goals. Here are some quick calculations that will help you figure out your estimated caloric needs based on your training goals.

FOR LEANING DOWN

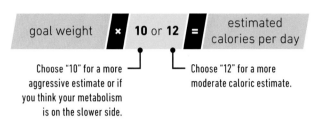

goal weight × 10 or 12 = estimated calories per day

Choose "10" for a more aggressive estimate or if you think your metabolism is on the slower side.

Choose "12" for a more moderate caloric estimate.

FOR MAINTENANCE OR BODY RECOMPOSITION (RECOMP)

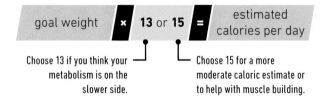

goal weight × 13 or 15 = estimated calories per day

Choose 13 if you think your metabolism is on the slower side.

Choose 15 for a more moderate caloric estimate or to help with muscle building.

FOR GAINING MUSCLE

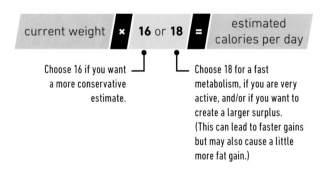

current weight × 16 or 18 = estimated calories per day

Choose 16 if you want a more conservative estimate.

Choose 18 for a fast metabolism, if you are very active, and/or if you want to create a larger surplus. (This can lead to faster gains but may also cause a little more fat gain.)

COMMON MACRO SPLITS

Below are some common macro splits. It's important to remember that your actual macro split is not nearly as important as your overall caloric intake. The only exception is when working toward gaining muscle as a slight caloric surplus of between 100 to 300 calories above maintenance calories is necessary. The surplus should come from carbs and protein as this will help minimize the amount of excess fat gain. If your goal is to lean down, you must be in a caloric deficit. You must be at or around maintenance calories to maintain or recomp.

Before choosing a split, think about what types of food you crave when you're hungry. If you reach for crunchy, sweet, or starchy foods, you may do better with the high-carb or balanced plans. If you reach for rich, creamy, or decadent foods when hungry, you may benefit more from the balanced plan or the lower carb plan.

HIGH-CARB PLAN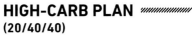
(20/40/40)

A high-carb plan is excellent for muscle gain and can provide energy for high-intensity activities. Higher carbs also aid in recovery, which means you can potentially train at a higher frequency than you would with other macro splits. Carbs are also protein-sparing, which means that your body will utilize them for energy rather than breaking down proteins. This plan works well for any goal.

DAILY MACRO SPLIT

FAT (20%): A low ratio of fats allows room for a greater ratio of carbs and protein. (Since fats are essential, it's not recommended to go below 20 percent.)

CARBS (40%): A high ratio of carbs is essential since the body needs carbs for fuel, recovery, and building or maintaining muscle.

PROTEIN (40%): You should consume 1–1.5 grams of protein per pound of goal body weight, per day. This ensures enhanced muscle building or muscle maintenance, and recovery. High-protein intake will also boost metabolism and improve feelings of satiety.

BALANCED FATS AND CARBS PLAN
(30/30/40)

This split offers an equal balance of fats and carbs, while keeping protein intake high for satiety and muscle maintenance, and for increasing metabolism. You may opt for this plan if you enjoy eating both carbs and fats or if you feel like you function well on either energy source. A balanced plan works well for any goal, though you may have better results with gaining muscle on the high-carb plan.

DAILY MACRO SPLIT

FAT (30%): A moderate fat intake may aid in recovery and also help promote feelings of satiety.

CARBS (30%): This split allows for enough carbs to boost energy levels and to aid in recovery from training.

PROTEIN (40%): Protein intake remains high to aid in muscle maintenance, recovery, and to aid a boosted metabolism. Aiming for around 1 gram per pound of your goal bodyweight is a good estimate.

LOWER CARB PLAN
(40/20/40)

This split is higher in fats and lower in carbs. If you feel like you don't digest carbs well or are sensitive to carbs, you may opt for this split. This split works well for recomping or for leaning down, but is not recommended for muscle gain.

DAILY MACRO SPLIT

FAT (40%): A higher dietary fat intake can help keep blood sugar levels steady and improve feelings of satiety.

CARBS (20%): While carb intake is lower, it should still allow for fueling your body both before and after training sessions.

PROTEIN (40%): Protein intake remains high to aid in muscle maintenance and recovery, and to also boost metabolism. Aim for around 1 gram per pound of your goal body weight.

EATING FOR MUSCLE GAIN

Good nutrition is the single most important factor when it comes to gaining muscle and changing body composition. You need to ensure that you're getting enough whole-food protein, carbs, and good fats in your diet. The timing of meals is also important. It can help maintain energy levels, help with recovery from training, and prevent overeating later in the day. Eating every few hours can prevent muscle loss, or *catabolism*. Eating to gain muscle can seem like a complicated task, but it doesn't have to be. Let's look at a few key factors that will greatly improve your success. The first step is deciding if your goal is body recomposition (recomping) by building muscle while also cutting fat or if it's strictly building muscle. If you're recomping, you'll be eating at maintenance calories, which means you'll be eating around the same number of calories that you burn each day. The result of this will be simultaneous fat loss and muscle gain. Recomping is a much slower process than muscle gain, but you won't need to go through separate "clean bulk" or "fat loss" phases, which means you can be generally more comfortable with your appearance throughout the process. If your goal is strictly gaining muscle, you'll be eating at a slight caloric surplus. This surplus can be anywhere between 100 to 300 calories beyond what you burn each day. This will allow the body to gain muscle at a much faster rate than recomping. A good way to think of it is as if you're building a house. Many materials are needed to create this new structure. If materials arrive daily, the house is built quickly. If you must go out and repurpose materials from other locations, the build is going to take longer.

DETERMINING MAINTENANCE CALORIES

You can estimate your maintenance calories by calculating your basal metabolic rate, or BMR, and then adding calories based on your activity level. (Calculator.net has a simple tool for figuring this out. I recommend estimating your activity level a bit lower than what the chart suggests.) Most people tend to overestimate how active they are, and it's easier to add calories based on progress than to start your program with excess fat gain. Another way to determine maintenance calories is to keep a food log and track your weight and measurements every week or every other week. This will give you a better idea of how to adjust your caloric intake to gain muscle. Once you've determined your maintenance calories, add 100 to 300 calories to your daily intake. It's best to add these calories in the form of carbs and protein. Aim to eat a bit more both before and after training.

PRE- AND POST-WORKOUT MEAL TIMING

To maximize muscle gain success, you'll need to focus most of your efforts on what you eat both before and after training. These pre- and post-workout meals will give you the fuel you need to train and also the nourishment you need for muscle gain and muscle recovery. Both of these meals should be high in carbs, moderate in protein, low in fat, and low in fiber. This formula will make it easier for your body to digest these meals and assimilate the nutrients. So why should these meals be low fat and low fiber? Fats and fiber slow down digestion. At any other time of the day this would aid in satiety, but meals higher in fats and fiber can delay absorption of nutrients that can help with muscle recovery, muscle repair, and the replenishment of energy stores. Fats are also an essential macronutrient for hormone production, cellular function, and the absorption of vitamins. And because fats provide energy, they must be included in any meal plan. If your goal is to gain muscle, your overall fat intake should be low, but not less than 20 percent of your body weight.

Your pre-workout meal should contain a complex carb like rice, sweet potato, potato, or oatmeal, and a protein such as any lean meat, fish, egg whites, or a lean vegetarian protein source. This meal should be consumed 1 to 2 hours before training.

Your post-workout meal works best if it's consumed within 1 hour of training. This meal can contain faster-digesting carbs like fruit, white rice, rice cakes, or quick oats. And if you incorporate protein shakes into your diet, a post-workout meal is a great time to drink one. Shakes are generally absorbed much faster than whole foods and can help replenish your energy stores more quickly. If you don't drink shakes, any lean source of protein will work well.

MAXIMIZING MUSCLE GAIN
WHILE MINIMIZING FAT GAIN

It's impossible to gain muscle without gaining some fat—it's just part of the process. It is possible, however, to minimize fat gain while still maximizing muscle gain. To do so, make sure your caloric surplus beyond your maintenance calories is modest: 100 to 300 calories per day tends to work for most people. However, you may need to adjust this number based on your weekly or biweekly progress. Taking measurements and weighing in once per week can be so helpful. If your weight increases by more than 0.5 percent of your body weight each week or if your waist measurement increases more than your other measurements, you will need to reduce your daily caloric intake. If your weight and measurements don't change, you'll need to increase your caloric intake. Aim for upward or downward adjustments of about 100 to 300 calories, and then give your body a week or two to gauge if the adjustments were sufficient or if you need to adjust further. Don't be afraid to adjust, as your body changes all the time.

The next factor for maximizing muscle gain while minimizing fat loss is making sure your caloric surplus is in the form of carbs and protein. Protein is not easily stored as body fat, even when it's eaten in excess. Carbs are a bit easier to store as body fat, but carbs also help prevent muscle loss, aid in recovery, and are protein-sparing, which means the body will burn carbs for energy instead of breaking down muscle. It also means that you can reduce protein intake slightly to allow for a higher carb intake. You will not want to consume your excess calories in fat calories as the body will easily store dietary fat as body fat. This happens with amazing efficiency, with around 97 percent of excess fat calories being stored as body fat! Each meal and snack should contain protein. Your pre- and post-workout meals will have the greatest amount of carbs and should be low fat (less than 5 to 7 grams). Keep in mind that you do need fats, but keeping the fats relatively low will give you more of a caloric budget for both carbs and protein.

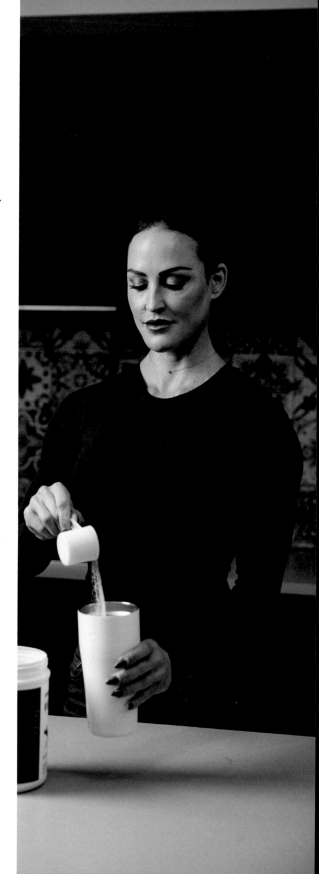

NUTRITION SUPPLEMENTS

Supplements can serve several different purposes: they can fill gaps in nutrition, boost performance and recovery, help with fat loss and improve body composition, and enhance overall health. With that said, there is a sea of products out there, so let's focus on the most-researched and proven supplements and their benefits.

WHEY PROTEIN

If you struggle to get enough protein in your diet or if you're just looking for a quick and convenient way to digest a post-workout snack, whey protein can be a great option. There are three types of whey protein: hydrolysate, isolate, and concentrate. Hydrolysate is the fastest-digesting form of whey protein, but it's also the most processed and most expensive. If you're lactose intolerant, hydrolysate may be the easiest on your stomach since it's usually lactose-free. (Check the label to be sure.) Isolate is the most popular form of whey protein; it's fast-digesting and reasonably priced. Relatively quick, but not nearly as quick as the first two options, is whey concentrate. Whey concentrate has a lower percentage of protein as it also contains some lactose and fats, which can slow down digestion.

If you can't stomach whey or if you eat a plant-based diet, there are other options. For omnivores, egg or beef protein is highly bioavailable, meaning that your body can utilize most of the protein in the serving. Vegans or vegetarians will likley want to choose a plant-based protein that has a complete amino acid profile. Just know that vegan protein sources tend to have lower bioavailability, meaning that it likely will require a larger serving size to ensure you're getting enough protein.

CREATINE MONOHYDRATE

The gold standard supplement for muscle and strength gains is creatine monohydrate. Creatine aids in recovery and can help you get more quality volume in each workout. It's one of the most well-studied supplements ever produced, and in addition to the athletic benefits, creatine can improve cognitive function and has added fat-loss benefits for athletes over 50. There are quite a few different types of creatine out there, but none are as thoroughly examined and as reasonably priced as creatine monohydrate.

It was once thought that you should try to get as much creatine into the muscle as quickly as possible by *loading,* or taking upward of 20 grams of creatine for the first 5 to 7 days when you first began taking it, but this is no longer believed to be the best approach. A dose of 2.5 grams per 100 pounds of bodyweight is sufficient. For some, creatine can cause stomach issues. If you experience this, try using 1 to 2 grams per day for 30 days to allow the creatine to be absorbed without excretion. It's important to note that creatine and caffeine should be taken at least one hour apart as caffeine can block creatine absorption. Adding it to your post-workout shake can be a good option.

GLUTAMINE

Glutamine can help improve recovery, enhance gut health and immunity, stabilize blood sugar, and potentially cut down on cravings. This super supplement can be taken before or after meals, and a typical dose is 2 to 5 grams per day, every day. After a workout, your muscles can be depleted of glutamine. Supplementing can replenish your body's glutamine stores and prevent muscle loss. The body can also be depleted of glutamine during times of high stress or illness, so this can be a handy supplement to keep in your stash.

ESSENTIAL AMINO ACIDS

Essential amino acids really shine if you're a vegan or vegetarian and you don't get enough protein, or if you're in a caloric deficit. The body can generate some amino acids, but not all. It needs 21 aminos to make up a complete protein, nine of which the body cannot generate alone. These nine amino acids are called *essential amino acids*. One of these amino acids, leucine, is responsible for increasing muscle protein synthesis or the process of creating new muscle from aminos. Animal sources of protein have plenty of leucine, which makes them a great option for muscle building. Many vegan sources of protein have limited amounts of essential amino acids. So if you are vegan, adding essential aminos to your routine can help you gain or maintain lean mass. If you're in a caloric deficit or dieting, aminos can help control appetite and prevent muscle breakdown. The same is true if you don't get enough dietary protein. Taking aminos before or after training is the most effective timing. A dose of 5 to 10 grams daily works well for most people.

CAFFEINE

If you're looking to boost energy, caffeine can be the answer. Additionally, caffeine can boost cognitive performance and workout performance, and some studies have shown that it can increase fat burning efficiency. Caffeine is a supplement to use with caution, though, as some people are sensitive to it and it can affect sleep quality. It can also interact with some medications and cause digestive disturbances, so be sure to thoroughly research it before incorporating it into your routine. The average dose is set by bodyweight and is typically between 1.4 to 2.7 milligrams per pound of bodyweight. The best time to incorporate caffeine is around 30 minutes before training.

FISH OIL

Chronic inflammation can often lead to disease, and the Standard American Diet (SAD) can exacerbate inflammation. One solution is to eat whole, unprocessed foods. To supplement these efforts, a good fish oil supplement will help boost your omega-3 levels and can help further reduce inflammation. Reducing inflammation reduces soreness, improves muscle gain by increasing muscle protein synthesis, and also enhances endurance capacity. Omega-3s found in fish oil include EPA and DHA, and the average daily dose is between 250 to 500 milligrams. A word of caution, though, fish oil can thin the blood.

SOME PRODUCTS TO AVOID

The supplement industry isn't heavily regulated, so you should avoid supplements that aren't certified. Look for supplements from third party-verified companies that include "certified safe for sport" or "informed choice" logos on their products to ensure quality and purity.

- ▸ Avoid generic multivitamins as the vitamins and minerals tend to be mostly man–made and the body doesn't recognize them, which often means the ingredients can simply pass through the body rather than being absorbed.
- ▸ Avoid supplements that claim to boost hormones. These can have the opposite effect and can throw the body out of balance.
- ▸ Steer clear of fat burners, especially those containing ingredients like yohimbe or rauwolscine (alpha-yohimbine). Negative side effects of fat burners can include dizziness, rapid heartbeat, nausea, and sleep disturbances.
- ▸ Avoid products that contain artificial colors like FD&C red or blue.
- ▸ Avoid products with fillers like titanium dioxide (a whitening agent) or potassium sorbate (a preservative) as these can potentially cause harm or irritation.

BUILDING YOUR HOME GYM

One of the really surprising things about training at home is that you don't need a huge space or a ton of equipment to mimic almost any exercise you can perform in a gym. However, you should do some planning before you ever invest in any equipment. Available space, budget, and versatility of equipment should all be carefully considered before you begin to build your home gym.

Keep in mind that you can still do the workouts in this book if your equipment differs slightly. Resistance bands with handles will work just as well as resistance bands with loops. And if you don't have a variety of dumbbells, check out the exercise variations to find an option that will work with what you have on hand. There's a good chance that there's a variation for every exercise that you can do with what you already have and still make progress. Certain pieces of equipment are necessary. An adjustable bench is needed to properly and safely perform many of the exercises. If budget is a concern, check out consignment shops, garage sales, or online classifieds—you can usually find great deals. If your goal is to build your ideal physique, make sure you have as many of the tools as possible in order to start building!

EQUIPMENT

This basic equipment will help you to not only get in a good workout, it will be enough to help you gain strength and build muscle.

ADJUSTABLE BENCH An adjustable bench is the perfect tool for training your muscles at various angles and ensuring that you're targeting the muscle fibers in a variety of ways to improve progress. The ideal bench will be adjustable from flat to 90 degrees, with incremental angles in between. If you're able to find a bench that adjusts to a decline, that's even better—you'll be able to perform additional exercises like hip thrusts and split squats. If you have a designated home gym area, a heavier bench can be a better option as it will be less likely than a lighter bench to slide or budge while you're using bands. If your training area must be packed away after each workout, a lighter bench with wheels can be a good choice.

DUMBBELLS A few sets of lighter dumbbells and a couple of heavier single dumbbells will enable you to train both upper- and lower-body muscles. Depending on your current level of strength, sets of 5-pound, 10-pound, and 15-pound dumbbells should

CHOOSING A SPACE

Before you invest in any equipment, you should determine how big of an area you'll need to devote to your training and if the equipment will all fit in the space. It's also a good idea to decide if your home gym can be in a space where equipment can be left out all the time. If this is the case, consider investing in heavier or sturdier equipment as it can last longer and will be a bit safer to use, and you won't have to pull the equipment out every time you want to train. If you need to tuck your home gym away after each use, consider purchasing lighter equipment that can easily be broken down and moved out of the way in a relatively short period of time.

The goal is to cut down on the number of obstacles that can get in the way of your training. Constantly lugging out and then stowing away equipment is a big reason why so many people give up when they're training at home. If you're able to devote space in a garage or spare bedroom to a home gym, you'll be one step closer to long-term success. If this isn't possible, don't worry. You can still be successful by creating a consistent routine; investing in lighter, more manageable equipment; and just committing to sticking with it for a few weeks. Your routine will become habit, and habit becomes a lifestyle over time. You've got this!

give you plenty of training options. For heavier single dumbbells, weights between 30 and 60 pounds can be good choices. When considering these heavier options, think about how much you're currently lifting for heavier compound movements like goblet squats and dumbbell deadlifts, and then consider purchasing a dumbbell that matches your current level of strength, along with a heavier dumbbell that will allow for gains in strength.

LOOP RESISTANCE BANDS A set of loop resistance bands will give you an almost unlimited assortment of training options. These bands make back-training at home possible, though you can also train pretty much every single muscle group with resistance bands. The lightest band can be used in an upper-body workout to add increased resistance to dumbbell exercises while the heaviest band is perfect for heavy hip thrusts or lat pull-downs. It's very important to identify a sturdy, anchored object to attach the bands to—this could be a staircase, a column, a heavy bench, or a heavy piece of furniture. A door attachment will enable you to secure your bands in a closed door jamb.

MINI BANDS Mini bands can add resistance to multiple leg and abs exercises. They usually come in sets of two to three and offer different levels of resistance. Look for stretchy fabric bands as they tend to last longer than the rubber mini bands.

STURDY BOOKS OR YOGA BLOCKS Increasing the range of motion in an exercise is a great way to increase difficulty without going heavier, and it can

also recruit different regions of a muscle. In a gym, weight plates are commonly used for this purpose, but at home you can improvise with old sturdy books or a yoga block.

YOGA MAT OR TOWEL For comfort, a yoga mat or towel is recommended for abs exercises or for any exercise where you're sitting or lying on the floor. A good yoga mat will provide an extra layer of cushion while you're performing the exercise and will prevent you from slipping on a hard surface. A towel will also provide some comfort, but it won't necessarily prevent you from slipping on a hard surface.

GLIDING DISKS OR PAPER PLATES Gliding disks or paper plates can take your leg and abs exercises to an entirely different level. Sliding floor curls, for example, are the perfect substitute for leg curls that otherwise would be done on a machine in the gym. You can do the same exercise on the floor by simply using paper plates or sliding disks.

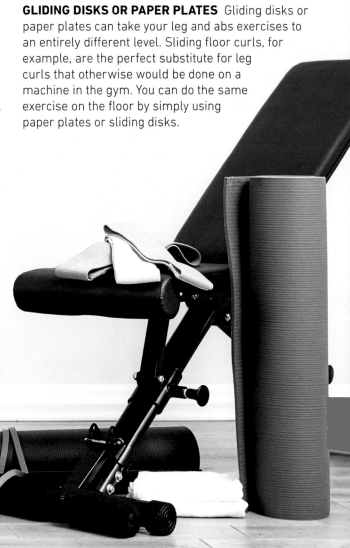

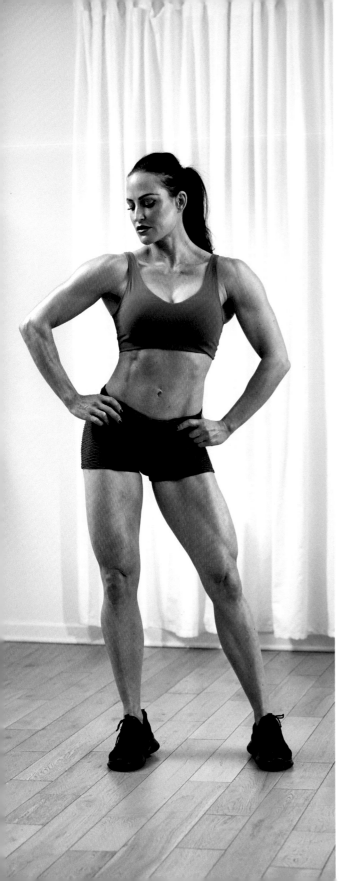

KNOW YOUR MUSCLES

You'll get the most from your lifts if you know the major muscle groups and how they work.

SHOULDERS

The shoulders are made up of three heads: front, side, and rear delts. The shoulder is the most mobile joint in the body and is one of the muscles responsible for moving the arms. Since the shoulder is so mobile, it can be trained through presses, raises, flyes, and upright rows, and with face pulls. Varying movements help ensure that all three heads are trained. To build width across the body, focus on the side delts; to improve upper-back width, focus on developing the rear delts.

BACK

The major muscle of the back is the latissimus dorsi, or *lats*. Developing the lats creates a beautiful V-taper. There are many smaller muscles of the back, including the trapezius, rhomboids, and teres. These upper-back muscles create dimension and width, which can make the waist appear smaller. The back is involved in all upper-body pulling movements, along with big compound lower-body movements like the deadlift and the squat.

CHEST

The main chest muscle is the pectoralis major, or *pecs,* which are divided into the upper and lower pecs. Chest muscles are used to move the arms across the body in upward and downward directions. They're also involved in flexion, which is the bending of a joint; raising the arm forward and upward (flexion at the shoulder joint); and internal rotation of the arms. (Tossing a ball with an underhand throw is an example of this.) You can target the chest with pressing movements and flyes. In this book, the focus will be a bit more on the upper chest as this can work to fill out the upper body and also tie the shoulders in with the rest of your physique.

BICEPS

The biceps brachii, or *biceps,* is responsible for flexing the lower arm toward the upper arm. The biceps has two heads: short and long. Performing a variety of curls and upper-body pulling movements will train and develop them well.

TRICEPS

The triceps brachii, or *triceps,* extends and retracts the forearm. The triceps stabilizes the shoulder and is divided into three heads: long, lateral, and medial. Push-downs, overhead extensions, kick-backs, and presses are all movements needed to fully develop the triceps.

ABDOMINALS

The abdominals, or *abs,* aren't just for looks. These hardworking muscles stabilize and support the upper body and help protect the spine. Abdominals are comprised of four main muscles: internal obliques, external obliques, rectus abdominis (also known as the six-pack), and transverse abdominis (TVA). The TVA acts as an internal girdle, and by training the TVA with planks and vacuums, you can reduce your waist circumference. Developing a six-pack can be achieved by performing abs exercises and reducing overall body-fat levels.

HAMSTRINGS

Hamstring muscles serve several purposes: extending the hip, flexing the knee, and rotating the lower leg when the knee is bent. The hamstrings are comprised of three muscles: biceps femoris, semitendinosus, and semimembranosus. Since the hamstrings are responsible for several movement patterns, they must be trained accordingly. Sliding leg curls, stiff-legged deadlifts and other lower-body compound movements can help develop all three hamstring muscles.

GLUTES

The largest and strongest muscles in the body are the glutes: gluteus maximus, gluteus medius, and gluteus minimus. Glutes stabilize the body, extend the hips, move the thighs, and rotate the thighs. Walking, sitting, standing, running—almost every activity involves the glutes. Well-developed glutes increase overall strength, speed, and power. Exercises like hip thrusts, squats, lunges, deadlifts, and even standing upper-body exercises will recruit the glutes.

CALVES

Calves move the feet, allow you to jump, and enable you to rotate your ankles. Calves are comprised of two muscles: the soleus and the gastrocnemius. The largest of the two—the gastrocnemius—is trained with straight-leg exercises like calf raises while seated calf raises target the soleus.

MUSCLE CHARTS

Understanding the basic musculature in your body is an essential part of being a bodybuilder.

This guide will help you learn where the major muscle groups in the body are located, as well as where smaller muscles are located within the larger muscle groups.

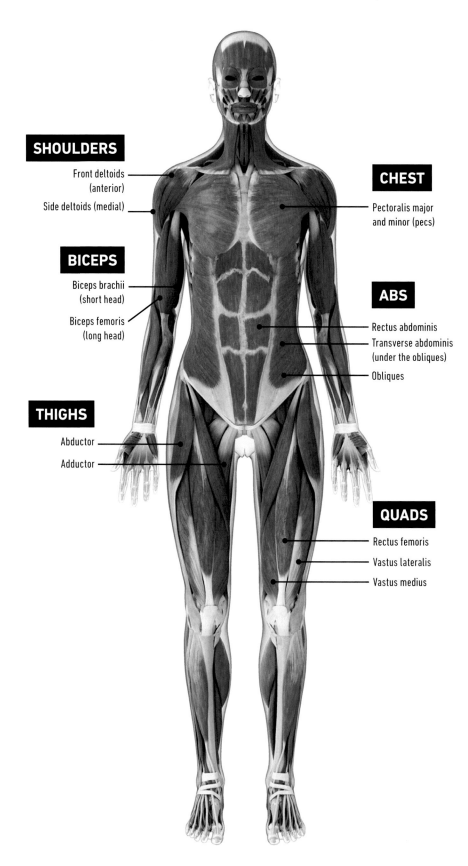

SHOULDERS

Front deltoids (anterior)

Side deltoids (medial)

BICEPS

Biceps brachii (short head)

Biceps femoris (long head)

THIGHS

Abductor

Adductor

CHEST

Pectoralis major and minor (pecs)

ABS

Rectus abdominis

Transverse abdominis (under the obliques)

Obliques

QUADS

Rectus femoris

Vastus lateralis

Vastus medius

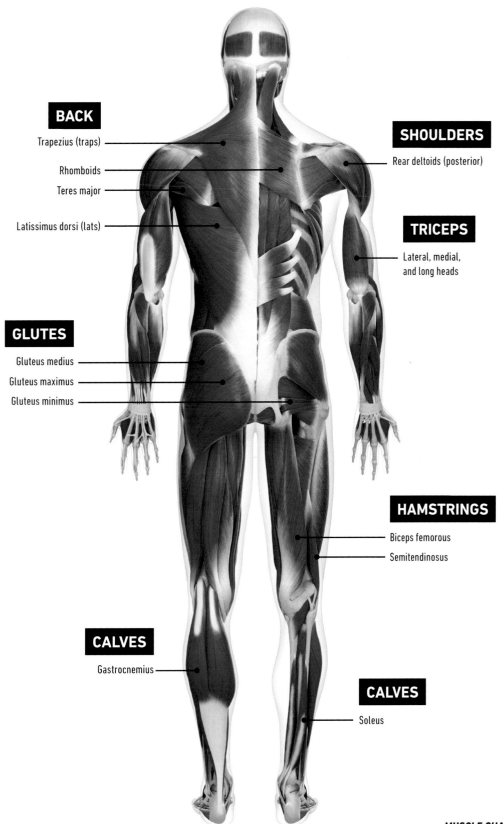

BACK

Trapezius (traps)

Rhomboids

Teres major

Latissimus dorsi (lats)

SHOULDERS

Rear deltoids (posterior)

TRICEPS

Lateral, medial, and long heads

GLUTES

Gluteus medius

Gluteus maximus

Gluteus minimus

HAMSTRINGS

Biceps femorous

Semitendinosus

CALVES

Gastrocnemius

CALVES

Soleus

TIPS FOR TRAINING AT HOME

Training at home can be a little more challenging than training at a gym, but with some forethought and planning, you'll be able to create the perfect atmosphere for success.

CREATE YOUR "GYM" SPACE

Consider where you will train. If you have a dedicated room where you can create a home gym, it can help cut out potential excuses and make it easier to get your workouts in. It's okay if you don't have a dedicated gym space—many people simply stow away their equipment when they're not using it. If you do this, just be sure to have a designated training area and quick methods for setting up and putting away your equipment. As you're curating your training space, think about your goals. If your goal is to gain muscle, you may need more sets of dumbbells and heavier resistance bands. If your goal is to lean down, you may need more open space for HIIT activities and more cardio-based activities like jumping rope or using kettlebells.

SET YOUR ROUTINE

Training around the same time each day has massive benefits—this holds true even if you're training just a few times each week. Keeping consistent schedules creates structure and encourages the creation of habits. Many people find that they need to work hard to adhere to a program for the first two to three weeks, but after that it becomes easier. If you can stick to your training schedule for a little over two months, you will have developed a lasting habit! You'll be more likely to maintain a healthy weight year-round and much less likely to miss your workouts.

START SMALL AND HAVE FUN!

If you haven't worked out in a while or if you're a beginner, start with less volume and lighter weights. Focus on proper form and ease into the habit of working out. By doing so you won't make yourself incredibly sore and be unable to train for days afterward. If you push yourself too hard in the beginning, you'll be less likely to stick with it. A benefit to beginning a new workout plan is that you'll enjoy "newbie gains," which means you won't need as much volume or weight to see results initially. Even if you are advanced, you can still see great progress by changing your routine, focusing on mind-muscle connection, and keeping constant tension on the muscles.

Have fun! If you condition yourself to view working out as punishment, you're much less likely to stick with it. Make sure your goals are clear, objective, and not rooted in self-judgment. Visualize your ideal body and how it moves, looks, and feels. Each workout will bring you closer to your ideal physique, which will help you create excitement around training.

ADJUST REP RANGES AND ADD RESISTANCE AS NEEDED

Muscle gains can be made in reps ranging anywhere from 5 to 30. This means that if you have limited equipment available, you can always add reps to the exercises and still see results. A good rule of thumb is to push each set to between 1 and 4 reps shy of failure. You can also add resistance bands to many exercises to create more tension on the muscles that very closely mimics training on machines or with cables. It's an easy and low-cost way to continue to make progress with limited equipment. Be honest with yourself about the effort you're putting in; if your workouts aren't challenging, you will not see the results you're hoping for. If you're just starting out, don't worry! Just do your best and be consistent! You'll be more able to gauge intensity as you gain more experience with training.

TRACK WORKOUTS AND TRACK PROGRESS

Keep a detailed log of sets and reps for each exercise, along with notes regarding the techniques you've used. By doing this, you'll be able to successfully keep tabs on your overall volume as well as any adjustments you've made in previous workouts. When working through a program, a 10 percent increase in overall volume each week will typically lead to progress. An easy-to-follow structure would be to follow a program for 4 to 6 weeks, increasing the difficulty or volume each week, and then taking a week to allow your body to rest and reset (also called a *deload week*). After taking a week off from training, your body will be more sensitive to training. This will allow you to begin your new plan at a lower overall lifting volume than you finished the last plan with, and you'll still make progress!

It's tough to know if you've made progress by looking in the mirror each day. Daily changes are so small that you won't be able to notice them, but you will be able to notice improvements by taking progress photos and placing them side by side or by taking measurements. If possible, try doing both; the more data you can collect, the better able you will be to adjust and troubleshoot. Make sure you're measuring and taking photos the same way each time so you'll be able to easily compare before and after shots.

You can also use a scale, but you shouldn't overly rely on it. Scales don't tell the whole story—gaining muscle mass and losing body fat will result in little-to-no change on the scale, but your body composition and appearance will change dramatically.

MAKE SURE YOUR TRAINING ENVIRONMENT ALIGNS WITH YOUR GOALS

It's important that your training environment aligns with your goals. If you want to step on a bodybuilding stage in the future, you should invest in heavier dumbbells and solid equipment. You may even want to have a permanent home gym as dragging out heavy equipment on a daily basis can create obstacles to training. Even if you have no desire to compete on a stage, a training environment that aligns with your goals will still be important to your success. You should decide how you like to train! Whether it's in a quiet zen environment or with music blasting, a space that's free of distractions will encourage you to get your workouts in. If it's not possible to eliminate distractions, work to limit them by turning off the television, using headphones, or scheduling your workouts when you know you won't be interrupted. A small amount of planning will set you up for big success!

///// **TIP** /////
Ultimately, success in creating your ideal physique comes from consistency. Many people will talk about motivation—but it's more than just that! It's about commitment to yourself and to your goals. So make a commitment to build your best. You're worth it!

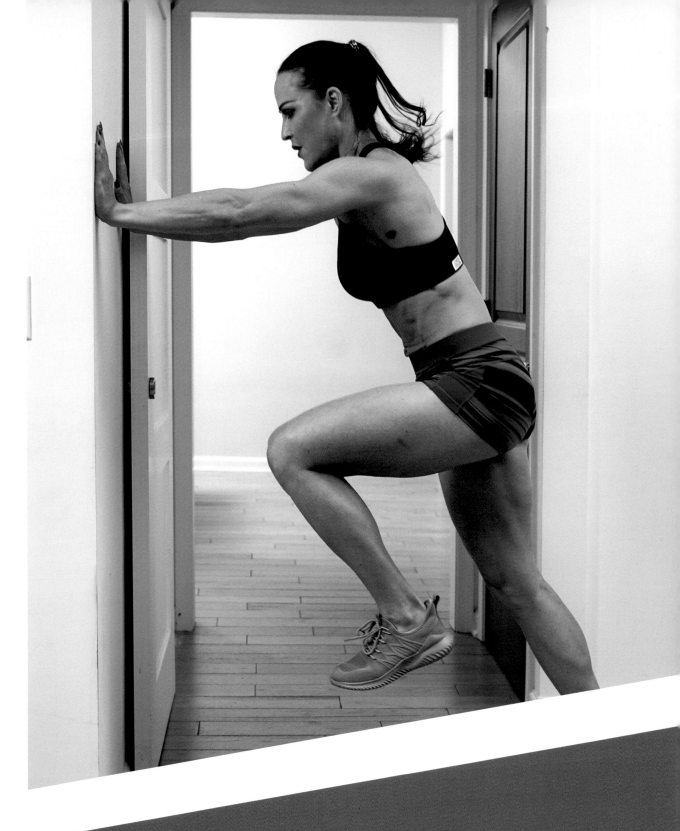

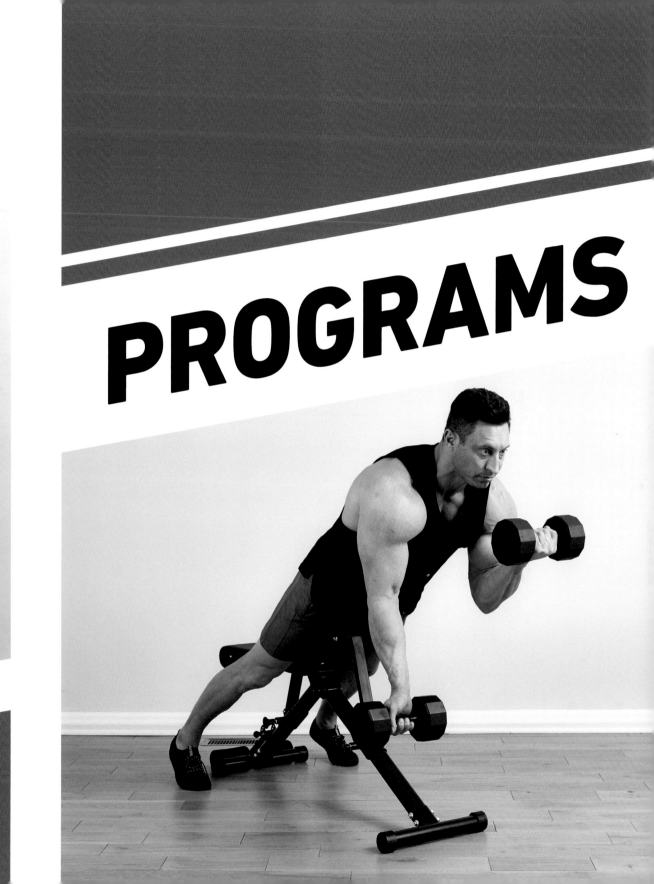

PROGRAMS

CHOOSING A TRAINING PROGRAM

Choosing a training program can seem overwhelming. So if you're wondering what program is best for you, just keep reading: I'll simplify things and help you come up with a solid game plan. When it comes to training, there are hundreds, if not thousands, of ways to accomplish your training goals, and that's a good thing! It gives you the ability to change your workouts every few weeks, which will decrease the chances of you plateauing while also keeping workouts fresh and fun. Whenever you do decide to change programs, just return to this section to ensure your new program aligns with your training goals.

DEFINE AND PRIORITIZE YOUR TRAINING GOALS

The first step is to define your training goals. Is your goal to be leaner, stronger, more athletic, more muscular, or a mix of the four? Try to define three to four specific physique goals, and then consider each muscle group that will need to be trained in order to meet those goals. If you want to add more muscle, you'll need to define exactly where you want to add it. If you want to be leaner, you'll need to decide what areas you want to lean down. (It can be helpful to visualize your ideal physique in your mind as you make these decisions.) If you have more than one overall training goal, make sure the goals aren't divergent. For example, if you want to lean down, it will be very difficult for you to also get stronger as you get leaner. If you want to build cardio endurance, you'll likely have a difficult time gaining muscle mass. You can, however, gain endurance and get leaner, as these are converging goals.

Once you've defined your training goals, you'll need to prioritize them by figuring out which muscle or muscle groups are most important in terms of achieving your ideal physique and then deciding what improvements will yield the greatest impact for those muscle groups. For example, if you want a smaller waist, you can prioritize shoulder and upper-back work along with planks and vacuums. Your top goal should be the number one priority on day one of your program, your second most important goal should be emphasized on day two, followed by your third goal on day three, and so on.

It's also important to be realistic about how many days you can devote to training. If you know you can only train four days per week, don't start a program that requires six days of training per week. You can always add training days, so starting more conservatively will increase your chances for success. If you commit to more days per week than you can actually do, you may feel disappointed in your efforts and your motivation could suffer.

CHOOSE A PROGRAM

Once you've decided how many days per week you can train, you can choose one of the three options offered in the programs that follow. If you have multiple training goals but can only train four days per week, the 4-Day High-Frequency/Total Body Program is a great option. You'll hit target muscle groups in each training session, which can help you make progress more quickly. If your goal is to gain overall strength and get fitter, you may want to opt for either the 4-Day Upper-Lower Program or the 4-Day Push-Pull program.

If you have the ability to train five or six days per week, your options for targeting specific muscle groups are expanded as you'll have more days to split up priority muscle groups. The specialized splits programs offer dedicated workouts for each muscle group and include compound and isolation exercises. These programs can be good choices if you prefer to have a targeted goal in mind for each training day. If you like variety within each workout, you may want to opt for the 5-Day or 6-Day Push-Pull-Legs or High-Frequency programs. Push-Pull-Legs works on movement patterns versus specific muscles, so it can be a good choice if you like to focus on pressing moves on one day and then pulling moves on another. High-frequency training gives you total body workouts each session. And just like with the 4-day programs, you'll be hitting major muscle groups with each workout. This approach works well if you have multiple training goals or if you just enjoy training everything each time you work out.

There is no single right or wrong workout program. Any program can help you get closer to your goals. The key factors are choosing a realistic number of training days you can commit to each week and also shifting the training days to emphasize priority muscle groups at the beginning of each week (if you choose a specialized program).

MODIFYING THE PROGRAMS TO FIT YOUR NEEDS

Swapping days around in a prewritten program may seem a bit daunting, but it's possible if you follow a few rules.

When swapping a specialized day within a program, you should allow for 72 hours of recovery time between the same training days. So if you move your shoulder workout to a different day, make sure you also move the secondary shoulder workout to allow for proper recovery.

Don't plan to do HIIT two days in a row. You can always shift a HIIT workout without shifting a weight workout. And try not to do HIIT on leg days as it could be too much volume.

You can also move Push-Pull-Leg days around. You could potentially do legs, then pull, then push, but

you should allow 72 hours of recovery time between the first pull day and the second pull day. The same rule applies for for push days.

High-Frequency days can be shifted around at your discretion since the volume for each muscle group is relatively low, which means you can still train on back-to-back days.

PRIORITIZE THE MOST EFFECTIVE EXERCISES

In addition to shifting training days around to emphasize priority muscle groups, you can also shift exercises around within workouts. As a general rule for strength and power training, compound or more difficult movements should come at the beginning of workouts unless you're training for aesthetics, in which case you won't be going as heavy. As you move through your workouts, keep track of the exercises performed, weights lifted, and any modifications you make to the exercises. Add notes on which exercises are most effective for your priority muscle groups. By keeping a running rating system of exercises, you can easily shift exercises around in your workouts. I like using a scale from 1 to 10, with "10" being the exercise I feel targets the muscle best and "1" being the exercise I feel has the least impact. For example, if the goal is building shoulders, lateral raises may be a "10" for you while the shoulder press might only be a "5." Based on this, you can change the order of the exercises in the program so that your "9" and "10" exercises are prioritized at the beginning of each workout. This can help increase your rate of progress.

Training Program Notes

- Each day includes an optional Get Lean set for added calorie burn or an optional Gain Muscle set for added weight volume.

- AMRAP means as many reps as possible. When you see AMRAP listed in a program, it simply means you should perform the exercise to the point where you can no longer perform any more reps.

- A Superset combines two exercises into one set to train opposing muscle groups more efficiently. A Superset should feature alternating sets between each exercise.

- A Giant Set combines three exercises into one set, with one set of each exercise done in succession with the next and no rest in between sets.

4-DAY HIGH-FREQUENCY/TOTAL BODY PROGRAM

This program is great for those who can devote four days to training and want to focus on hitting each muscle group at least once per day. Research has shown that higher-frequency training can increase muscle protein synthesis, which leads to more muscle gains. If your goal is to lean down, this is still a good option as the plan features many compound movements, which can increase calorie burn and make for shorter workouts.

DAY 1

LEG ISOLATION/BACK

EXERCISE	SETS	REPS/ DURATION
Hip Thrust (p.76)	3	8
Goblet Squat (p.62)	3	10
Bench Reverse Hyper (p.86)	2	15
Quad Step-Up (p.70)	3	8/side
Supine Dumbbell Row (p.102)	2	8
Banded High-Row (p.94)	2	12
Reverse Flye (p.154)	2	15
GAIN MUSCLE (OPTIONAL)		
Dumbbell Pull-Over (p.98)	2	10
GET LEAN (OPTIONAL)		
Shadow Boxing (p.179)	5	30 sec.

DAY 2

ARM ISOLATION/SHOULDERS/CHEST/ABS

EXERCISE	SETS	REPS/DURATION
Single-Leg Bench-Assisted Squat (p.60)	3	10/side
Dumbbell Deadlift (p.74)	3	8
Straight-Leg Deadlift (p.72)	3	15
Seated Shoulder Press (p.144)	2	10
Dumbbell Incline Flye (p.122)	2	15
Lateral Raise (p.152)	2	10
Decline Push-Up (p.120)	2	AMRAP
GAIN MUSCLE (OPTIONAL)		
Wide-Grip Upright Row (p.146)	2	12
GET LEAN (OPTIONAL)		
Wall Sprint (p.181)		

ABS CIRCUIT

EXERCISE	SETS	REPS/DURATION
Vacuum (p.161)	4	10–15 sec.
X-Plank (p.160)	1	30–45 sec.
Hollow Hold (p.166)	1	30–45 sec.
Side Plank (p.168)	2	30–40 sec./ side

DAY 3 (REST)

LEG ISOLATION/BACK

DAY 4

EXERCISE	SETS	REPS/DURATION
Goblet Squat (p.62)	3	15
B-Stance Hip Thrust (p.77)	2	10/side
Reverse Nordic Curl (p.80)	2	8–10
Sliding Floor Curl (p.78)	2	8–10
Standing Calf Raise (p.88)	2	20
Banded Lat Pull-Down (p.92)	2	10
Banded Low Row (p.106)	2	20
Renegade Row (p.108)	2	20 (total)
GAIN MUSCLE (OPTIONAL)		
Goblet Squat (p.62)	2	15
GET LEAN (OPTIONAL)		
Dumbbell Swing (p.180)	5	15

LEG ISOLATION/SHOULDERS/CHEST/ABS

DAY 4

EXERCISE	SETS	REPS/DURATION
Spanish Squat (p.84)	3	20
Heel-Elevated Hack Squat (p.68)	3	12
Dumbbell Good Morning (p.82)	2	12
Y-Press (p.145)	3	12
Band Pull Apart (p.155)	2	20
Dumbbell Squeeze Press (p.119)	2	12
SUPERSET		
Bench Dip (p.130)	2	AMRAP
Standing Biceps Curl (p.132)	2	15
GAIN MUSCLE (OPTIONAL)		
Dumbbell Incline Bench Press (p.116) Lateral Raise (p.152)	2	8–10
GET LEAN (OPTIONAL)		
Incline Mountain Climber (p.186)	4	40 sec.

ABS CIRCUIT

EXERCISE	SETS	REPS/DURATION
Vacuum (p.161)	4	10–15 sec.
Knee-Up (p.164)	2	40 reps
V-Up (p.165)	2	20 reps
Banded Bicycle (p.167)	2	40 total

DAY 6 (REST)

DAY 7 (REST)

4-DAY PUSH-PULL PROGRAM

This plan differs from the traditional bodybuilder's split in that you'll focus more on specific movements rather than targeting specific muscle groups for each workout. This will allow you to not only overcome plateaus but also hit each muscle group twice per week. Stimulating the muscles more frequently can increase muscle-protein synthesis, which can lead to more muscle gains. This can be especially important when you can only devote 4 days per week to training. This plan is a good choice whether your goal is to gain muscle, maintain muscle, or lean down.

DAY 1

HEAVY PULL

EXERCISE	SETS	REPS/DURATION
Dumbbell Deadlift (p.74)	3	8
Hip Thrust (p.76)	3	10
Sliding Floor Curl (p.78)	3	8–10
Supine Dumbbell Row (p.102)	3	10
Banded Lat Pull-Down (p.92)	3	10
Wide-Grip Upright Row (p.146)	3	12
Banded Biceps Curl (p.134)	3	12
GAIN MUSCLE (OPTIONAL)		
Yates Row (p.100)	2	10
GET LEAN (OPTIONAL)		
Renegade Row (p.108)	5	30 sec.

DAY 2

HEAVY PUSH/ABS

EXERCISE	SETS	REPS/DURATION
Goblet Spanish Squat (p.85)	3	10
Heel-Elevated Hack Squat (p.68)	3	8
Y-Press (p.145)	3	8–10
Dumbbell Bench Press (p.114)	3	10
Dumbbell Squeeze Press (p.119)	3	10
Bench Dip (p.130)	3	10–12
Dumbbell Skullcrusher (p.138)	3	10
GAIN MUSCLE (OPTIONAL)		
Single-Leg Bench-Assisted Squat (p.60)	2	8/side
GET LEAN (OPTIONAL)		
Burpee (p.176)	5	15 sec.

ABS CIRCUIT

EXERCISE	SETS	REPS/DURATION
Vacuum (p.161)	4	10–15 sec.
Banded Crunch (p.162)	3	15–20
Banded Bicycle (p.167)	2	40 (total)
Toe Toucher (p.170)	3	20–25

DAY 3 (REST)

DAY 4

LIGHT PULL/ABS

EXERCISE	SETS	REPS/DURATION
Straight Leg Deadlift (p.72)	3	15
Bench Reverse Hyper (p.86)	3	15
Single-Arm Side Pull-Down (p.110)	3	12/side
Dumbbell Pull-Over (p.98)	3	15
Dumbbell Face Pull (p.148)	3	15
Spider Curl (p.136)	3	15
Standing Biceps Curl (p.132)	3	20
GAIN MUSCLE (OPTIONAL)		
Band Pull Apart (p.155)	2	20
GET LEAN (OPTIONAL)		
Incline Mountain Climber (p.186)	5	30 sec.

ABS CIRCUIT

EXERCISE	SETS	REPS/DURATION
Vacuum (p.161)	4	10–15 sec.
V-Up (p.165)	2	12–15
Side Plank (p.168)	2	30 sec./side

DAY 5

LIGHT PUSH

EXERCISE	SETS	REPS/DURATION
Quad Step-Up (p.70)	3	8–10/side
Cossack Squat (p.64)	3	10/side
Reverse Nordic Curl (p.80)	3	12–15
Seated Shoulder Press (p.144)	3	15
Lateral Raise (p.152)	3	20
Incline Push-Up (p.121)	3	15–18
Dumbbell Incline Flye (p.122)	3	20
GAIN MUSCLE (OPTIONAL)		
Dumbbell Press-Out (p.150)	2	12–15
GET LEAN (OPTIONAL)		
High Knees (p.178)	3	20 sec. (3x)

DAY 6 (REST)

DAY 7 (REST)

4-DAY UPPER-LOWER PROGRAM

If you only have four days per week to train, the upper-lower split in this program can effectively target all muscle groups, allowing for both strength and size gains. If your goal is to lean down, the two lower-body days will greatly increase calorie burn. Having a couple of days off per week decreases the chances of overuse injuries and can fit better into a busy schedule.

DAY 1

LOWER BODY

EXERCISE	SETS	REPS/DURATION
Goblet Skater Squat (p.163)	4	8
Mini-Band Straight-Leg Deadlift (p.73)	4	10
Bulgarian Split Squat (p.66)	3	8–10/side
Incline Bench Reverse Hyper (p.87)	3	10
Standing Calf Raise (p.88)	3	15
SUPERSET		
Reverse Nordic Curl (p.80)	3	12
Sliding Floor Curl (p.78)	3	12
GAIN MUSCLE (OPTIONAL)		
Dumbbell Deadlift (p.74)	2	15
GET LEAN (OPTIONAL)		
Pop Squat (p.182)	3	30 sec.

DAY 2

UPPER BODY/ABS

EXERCISE	SETS	REPS/DURATION
Seated Shoulder Press (p.144)	4	8
Seated Banded Row (p.96)	4	12
Banded Lateral Raise (p.153)	3	12
Banded Upright Row (p.147)	3	10
Banded Reverse Flye (p.155)	3	12
SUPERSET		
Incline Bench Skullcrusher (p.139)	3	12
Spider Curl (p.136)	3	12
GAIN MUSCLE (OPTIONAL)		
Bus Driver (p.156)	2	20 (total)
GET LEAN (OPTIONAL)		
Dumbbell Swing (p.180)	4	15

AB CIRCUIT

EXERCISE	SETS	REPS/DURATION
Vacuum (p.161)	3	AMRAP
Banded Crunch (p.162)	3	20
Side Plank (p.168)	2	30–40 sec./side

DAY 4

LOWER BODY //

EXERCISE	SETS	REPS/DURATION
Dumbbell Sumo Deadlift (p.75)	4	15
B-Stance Hip Thrust (p.77)	4	8/side
Offset Bulgarian Split Squat (p.67)	3	10/side
SUPERSET		
Quad Step-Up (p.70)	3	8/side
Lateral Lunge (p.65)	3	8
SUPERSET		
Heel-Elevated Hack Squat (p.68)	3	15
Dumbbell Good Morning (p.82)	3	15
Seated Dumbbell Calf Raise (p.89)	1	20/side
GAIN MUSCLE (OPTIONAL)		
Goblet Spanish Squat (p.85)	2	15
GET LEAN (OPTIONAL)		
Wall Sprint (p.181)	4	30 sec.

DAY 5

UPPER BODY/ABS //

EXERCISE	SETS	REPS/DURATION
Dumbbell Incline Bench Press (p.116)	4	10
Supine Dumbbell Row (p.102)	4	8
SUPERSET		
Dumbbell Incline Flye (p.122)	3	12
Incline Bench Skullcrusher (p.139)	3	15
SUPERSET		
Banded High Row (p.94)	3	15
Banded Biceps Curl (p.134)	3	15
SUPERSET		
Incline Push-Up (p.121)	3	10–12
Lateral Raise (p.152)	3	15
GAIN MUSCLE (OPTIONAL)		
Dumbbell Partial Rep Curl (p.133)	2	AMRAP
GET LEAN (OPTIONAL)		
Shadow Boxing (p.179)	5	30 sec.

ABS CIRCUIT ///

EXERCISE	SETS	REPS/DURATION
Vacuum (p.161)	4	10–15 sec.
X-Plank (p.160)	1	30–45 sec.
Knee-Up (p.164)	2	20
Toe Toucher (p.170)	2	20–25
Dead Bug (p.166)	2	30/side

5-DAY PUSH-PULL-LEGS PROGRAM

This plan focuses on movements and is especially good for those who are looking to build upper-body and maintain lower-body muscle, as four of the training days are dedicated to upper-body training. Each day will have a specific focus. For example, Day 1 is primarily for back. You will find biceps work on back-focused days and back work on biceps-focused days. This allows for greater frequency in training and for the opportunity to make faster gains.

DAY 1

PULL (BACK)

EXERCISE	SETS	REPS/DURATION
Supine Dumbbell Row (p.102)	3	10
Dumbbell Pull-Over (p.98)	3	10
Banded High Row (p.94)	3	12
SUPERSET		
Yates Row (p.100)	3	10
Dumbbell Pull-Over (p.98)	3	12
SUPERSET		
Banded Lat Pull-Down (p.92)	3	12
Banded Biceps Curl (p.134)	3	10
GAIN MUSCLE (OPTIONAL)		
Single-Arm Dumbbell Row (p.104)	2	10/side
GET LEAN (OPTIONAL)		
Wall Sprint (p.181)	5	30 sec.

DAY 2

PUSH (SHOULDERS, CHEST, AND ABS)

EXERCISE	SETS	REPS/DURATION
Y-Press (p.145)	3	AMRAP
Banded Bench Press (p.115)	3	8
Lateral Raise (p.152)	3	10
SUPERSET		
Dumbbell Incline Flye (p.122)	3	10
Incline Bench Skullcrusher (p.139)	3	12
SUPERSET		
Bench Dip (p.130)	3	10–12
Triceps Kickback (p.128)	3	15
GAIN MUSCLE (OPTIONAL)		
Dumbbell Press-Out (p.150)	2	8–10
GET LEAN (OPTIONAL)		
Dumbbell Thruster (p.187)	3	15

ABS CIRCUIT (ISOMETRIC)

EXERCISE	SETS	REPS/DURATION
Vacuum (p.161)	4	10–15 sec.
X-Plank (p.160)	2	40–50 sec.
Hollow Hold (p.166)	2	40–50 sec.
Side Plank (p.168)	1	30–40 sec./ side

DAY 3

LEGS

EXERCISE	SETS	REPS/DURATION
Dumbbell Deadlift (p.74)	4	8
Hip Thrust (p.76)	3	15
Straight-Leg Deadlift (p.72)	3	12
Standing Calf Raise (p.88)	3	20
SUPERSET		
Goblet Squat (p.62)	3	10
Bench Reverse Hyper (p.86)	3	12
SUPERSET		
Reverse Nordic Curl (p.80)	3	10–12
Sliding Floor Curl (p.78)	3	8–10
GAIN MUSCLE (OPTIONAL)		
Goblet Spanish Squat (p.85)	2	15
GET LEAN (OPTIONAL)		
Dumbbell Swing (p.180)	3	12–15

DAY 4

PULL (BICEPS AND ABS)

EXERCISE	SETS	REPS/DURATION
Banded Low Row (p.106)	3	12
Banded Lat Pull-Down (p.92)	3	15
Yates Row (p.100)	3	12
SUPERSET		
Wide-Grip Upright Row (p.146)	3	8
Spider Curl (p.136)	3	8–10
Banded Biceps Curl (p.134)	3	20
GAIN MUSCLE (OPTIONAL)		
Cross-Body Curl (p.133)	2	10/side
GET LEAN (OPTIONAL)		
Renegade Row (p.108)	4	30 sec.

ABS CIRCUIT

EXERCISE	SETS	REPS/DURATION
Vacuum (p.161)	4	10–15 sec.
Reverse Crunch Against a Wall (p.171)	2	15–20
Knee-Up (p.164)	2	20–25
Toe Toucher (p.170)	2	15–20

DAY 5

PUSH (TRICEPS)

EXERCISE	SETS	REPS/DURATION
Incline Push-Up (p.121)	3	AMRAP
Y-Press (p.145)	3	20
Dumbbell Incline Bench Press (p.116)	3	15
SUPERSET		
Reverse Flye (p.154)	3	15
Incline Bench Triceps Kickback (p.129)	3	12
SUPERSET		
Bus Driver (p.156)	3	20 (total)
Wide-Grip Triceps Push-Down (p.141)	3	12
GAIN MUSCLE (OPTIONAL)		
Feet-Elevated Bench Dip (p.131)	2	8–10
GET LEAN (OPTIONAL)		
Wall Sprint (p.181)	5	15 sec.

DAY 6 (REST)

DAY 7 (REST)

5-DAY SPECIALIZED SPLIT PROGRAM

The specialized split gives more volume and focus to a particular muscle group each day. This split can be especially effective if you're looking for aesthetic improvements in your physique. The addition of a second leg day not only gives more focus to leg development but also enhances calorie burn. There is dedicated arm work on Day 5, but keep in mind that arms are trained with all upper-body pushing and pulling movements as well.

DAY 1 — LEGS (GLUTES AND HAMSTRINGS)

EXERCISE	SETS	REPS/DURATION
Dumbbell Deadlift (p.74)	4	8
B-Stance Hip Thrust (p.77)	3	10/side
Straight-Leg Deadlift (p.72)	3	12
SUPERSET		
Goblet Squat (p.62)	3	10
Dumbbell Good Morning (p.82)	3	12
SUPERSET		
Sliding Floor Curl (p.78)	3	10–12
Bulgarian Split Squat (p.66)	3	8/side
GAIN MUSCLE (OPTIONAL)		
Bench Reverse Hyper (p.86)	2	15
GET LEAN (OPTIONAL)		
Pop Squat (p.182)	4	30

DAY 2 — SHOULDERS

EXERCISE	SETS	REPS/DURATION
Banded Shoulder Press (p.145)	4	8
Wide-Grip Upright Row (p.146)	3	10
Reverse Flye (p.154)	3	12
SUPERSET		
Y-Press (p.145)	3	12
Lateral Raise (p.152)	3	10
SUPERSET		
Dumbbell Face Pull (p.148)	3	12
Dumbbell Press-Out (p.150)	3	10
GAIN MUSCLE (OPTIONAL)		
Band Pull Apart (p.155)	2	25–30
GET LEAN (OPTIONAL)		
Shadow Boxing (p.179)	5	30 sec.

DAY 3

BACK/ABS

EXERCISE	SETS	REPS/DURATION
Wide-Grip Pull-Down (p.93)	4	10–12
Banded Row (p.94) (pause reps)	3	10
Single-Arm Side Pull-Down (p.110)	3	8/side
SUPERSET		
Banded High Row (p.94)	3	10
Banded Straight Arm Push-Down (p.99)	3	12
SUPERSET		
Supine Dumbbell Row (p.102)	3	10
Incline Dumbbell Pull-Over (p.99)	3	12
GAIN MUSCLE (OPTIONAL)		
Banded Low Row (p.106)	2	10
GET LEAN (OPTIONAL)		
Renegade Row (p.108)	3	24 (total)

ABS CIRCUIT

EXERCISE	SETS	REPS/DURATION
Vacuum (p.161)	4	AMRAP
Banded Crunch (p.162)	2	20–25
Banded Curl-Up (p.163)	2	15–20
Toe Toucher (p.170)	2	25–30
Hollow Hold (p.166)	2	30–40 sec.

DAY 4

LEGS (QUADS AND CALVES)

EXERCISE	SETS	REPS/DURATION
Goblet Spanish Squat (p.85)	4	12
Heel-Elevated Hack Squat (p.68)	3	10
Quad Step-Up (p.70)	3	8/side
SUPERSET		
Offset Bulgarian Split Squat (p.67)	3	8/side
Single-Leg Bench-Assisted Squat (p.60)	3	8/side
SUPERSET		
Reverse Nordic Curl (p.80)	3	10–15
Standing Calf Raise (p.88)	3	20
GAIN MUSCLE (OPTIONAL)		
Dumbbell Sumo Deadlift (p.75)	2	12
GET LEAN (OPTIONAL)		
Dynamic Step-Up (p.183)	2	16 (total)

DAY 5

CHEST/ARMS/

EXERCISE	SETS	REPS/DURATION
Dumbbell Bench Press (p.114)	4	10
Decline Push-Up (p.120)	3	AMRAP
Banded Cross-Body Chest Press (p.124)	3	10/side
GIANT SET		
Dumbbell Incline Flye (p.122)	3	12
Incline Bench Skullcrusher (p.139)	3	12
Spider Curl (p.136)	3	12
GIANT SET		
Plyo Push-Up (p.184)	3	10–15
Wide-Grip Triceps Push-Down (p.141)	3	12
Banded Biceps Curl (p.134)	3	10
GAIN MUSCLE (OPTIONAL)		
Dumbbell Squeeze Press (p.119)	2	10
GET LEAN (OPTIONAL)		
Wall Sprint (p.181)	5	20 sec.

DAY 6 (REST)

DAY 7 (REST)

5-DAY
HIGH-FREQUENCY PROGRAM

This high-frequency plan targets most muscle groups each day, but at a much lower volume than a specialized split. This program can enhance muscle growth as you're stimulating the muscles almost every day. If you love variety and have always worked on traditional splits, this program can help with breaking through plateaus and can bring new life to a stale routine.

DAY 1

EXERCISE	SETS	REPS/DURATION
B-Stance Hip Thrust (p.77)	3	10 (each)
Goblet Squat (p.62)	3	12
Dumbbell Good Morning (p.82)	3	10
SUPERSET		
Reverse Nordic Curl (p.81)	2	12–15
Sliding Floor Curl (p.78)	2	12–15
Banded Lateral Raise (p.153)	3	8
Seated Shoulder Press (p.144)	2	12–15
GAIN MUSCLE (OPTIONAL)		
Dumbbell Press-Out (p.150)	2	10–12
GET LEAN (OPTIONAL)		
Incline Mountain Climber (p.186)	4	30 sec.

DAY 2

EXERCISE	SETS	REPS/DURATION
Quad Step-Up (p.70)	3	8/side
Dumbbell Deadlift (p.74)	3	12
SUPERSET		
Bench Reverse Hyper (p.86)	3	15
Standing Calf Raise (p.88)	3	20
SUPERSET		
Single-Arm Dumbbell Row (p.104)	2	10/side
Single-Arm Dumbbell Pull-Over (p.99)	2	10/side
Banded Incline Bench Press (p.117)	2	15
GAIN MUSCLE (OPTIONAL SUPERSET)		
Spider Curl (p.136)	2	12
Incline Bench Triceps Kickback (p.129)	2	12
GET LEAN (OPTIONAL)		
Dumbbell Thruster (p.187)	3	20

DAY 3

EXERCISE	SETS	REPS/DURATION
Spanish Squat (p.84)	3	15
Seated Dumbbell Calf Raise (p.89)	3	10/side
SUPERSET		
Banded Lat Pull-Down (p.92)	2	20
Banded Triceps Push-Down (p.140)	2	15
Y-Press (p.145)	3	10
Wide-Grip Upright Row (p.146)	3	12
Bench Dip (p.130)	2	10–12
GAIN MUSCLE (OPTIONAL)		
Dumbbell Incline Squeeze Press (p.118)	2	10
GET LEAN (OPTIONAL SUPERSET)		
Bear Crawl with Dumbbells (p.185)	3	15 sec.
Renegade Row (p.108)	3	15 sec.

ABS CIRCUIT

EXERCISE	SETS	REPS/DURATION
Banded Curl-Up (p.163)	1	15–20
Reverse Band Crunch (p.163)	1	15–20
Banded Bicycle (p.167)	1	30 (total)
Flutter Kick (p.166)	1	30 (total)

DAY 4

EXERCISE	SETS	REPS/DURATION
Bulgarian Split Squat (p.66)	3	8/side
Heel-Elevated Hack Squat (p.68)	3	12
Mini-Band Straight-Leg Deadlift (p.73)	3	15–18
Sliding Floor Curl (p.78)	2	10–12
Decline Push-Up (p.120)	3	6–8
Banded Reverse Flye (p.155)	2	12
Bus Driver (p.156)	2	20
GAIN MUSCLE (OPTIONAL)		
Yates Row (p.100)	2	15
GET LEAN (OPTIONAL)		
Incline Mountain Climber (p.186)	5	20 sec.

DAY 5

EXERCISE	SETS	REPS/DURATION
Hip Thrust (p.76)	3	20
Banded Pull-Through (p.83)	3	15
Dumbbell Deficit Deadlift (p.75)	2	12
SUPERSET		
Standing Calf Raise (p.88)	2	25
Lateral Lunge (p.65)	2	12/side
Banded Lat Pull-Down (p.92)	3	10
Dumbbell Press-Out (p.150)	2	15–18
GAIN MUSCLE (OPTIONAL)		
Banded Cross-Body Chest Press (p.124)	2	10/side
GET LEAN (OPTIONAL)		
Burpee (p.176)	2	10

ABS CIRCUIT

EXERCISE	SETS	REPS/DURATION
Vacuum (p.161)	3	AMRAP
X-Plank (p.160)	3	30–45 sec.
Lying Leg Raise (p.172)	3	12–15
Tuck Crunch (p.173)	3	15–18

DAY 6 (REST)

DAY 7 (REST)

6-DAY SPECIALIZED SPLIT PROGRAM

If you have six days to train per week and would like to have specific goals for each training day, this plan is a great choice. You'll be able to hit all muscle groups at least twice per week, which will not only accelerate progress but enhance overall calorie burn for the week as well. Whether your goal is to lean down, recomp, or gain muscle, you will see results by following this program. Be sure to track your food intake so that it aligns with your training goals.

DAY 1 — LEGS

EXERCISE	SETS	REPS/DURATION
SUPERSET		
Heel-Elevated Hack Squat (p.68)	3	8
Straight-Leg Deadlift (p.72)	3	12
SUPERSET		
Dumbbell Deficit Deadlift (p.75)	3	8
Bulgarian Split Squat (p.66)	3	8/side
SUPERSET		
Incline Bench Reverse Hyper (p.87)	3	12
Standing Calf Raise (p.88)	3	20
SUPERSET		
Reverse Nordic Curl (p.80)	2	12–14
Sliding Floor Curl (p.78)	2	12–14
GAIN MUSCLE (OPTIONAL)		
Cossack Squat (p.64)	2	8/side
GET LEAN (OPTIONAL)		
Dumbbell Thruster (p.187)	3	15

DAY 2 — BACK

EXERCISE	SETS	REPS/DURATION
SUPERSET		
Banded Lat Pull-Down (p.92)	3	8
Banded Straight-Arm Push-Down (p.99)	3	10
SUPERSET		
Single-Arm Dumbbell Row (p.104)	3	10
Dumbbell Pull-Over (p.98)	3	12
SUPERSET		
Banded Low Row (p.106)	3	12
Banded High Row (p.94)	3	12
Banded Face Pull (p.149)	3	12–14
GAIN MUSCLE (OPTIONAL)		
Supine Dumbbell Row (p.102)	2	12
GET LEAN (OPTIONAL)		
Burpee (p.176)	2	10–12/side

ABS CIRCUIT

EXERCISE	SETS	REPS/DURATION
Vacuum (p.161)	4	15–20 sec.
Side Plank with Abductor Lift (p.169)	2	20/side
High Plank Leg Lift (p.160)	2	20/side
Dead Bug (p.166)	2	15/side
GAIN MUSCLE (OPTIONAL)		
Supine Dumbbell Row (p.102)	2	12

DAY 3 — SHOULDERS

EXERCISE	SETS	REPS/DURATION
SUPERSET		
Seated Shoulder Press (p.144)	3	8
Wide-Grip Upright Row (p.146)	3	12
SUPERSET		
Lateral Raise (p.152)	3	14–16
Y-Press (p.145)	3	12–15
SUPERSET		
Dumbbell Press-Out (p.150)	3	12
Banded Upright Row (p.147)	3	12
Dumbbell Face Pull (p.148)	3	12–15

CONTINUES...

EXERCISE	SETS	REPS/DURATION
CIRCUIT		
Single Dumbbell Front Raise (p.157)	1	AMRAP
Reverse Flye (p.154)	1	AMRAP
Lateral Raise (p.152)	1	AMRAP
GAIN MUSCLE (OPTIONAL)		
Dumbbell Deficit Deadlift (p.75)	2	15
GET LEAN (OPTIONAL SUPERSET)		
Incline Mountain Climber (p.186)	5	15 sec.
Shadow Boxing (p.179)	5	15 sec.

DAY 4

LEGS

EXERCISE	SETS	REPS/DURATION
B-Stance Hip Thrust (p.77)	3	10/side
SUPERSET		
Goblet Squat (p.62)	3	8–10
Seated Dumbbell Calf Raise (p.89)	3	10/side
SUPERSET		
Goblet Spanish Squat (p.85)	3	12
Mini-Band Straight-Leg Deadlift (p.73)	3	12
SUPERSET		
Dumbbell Good Morning (p.82)	3	12–15
Bulgarian Split Squat (p.66)	3	8/side
SUPERSET		
Quad Step-Up (p.70)	2	8/side
Single-Leg Sliding Floor Curl (p.79)	2	6–8/side
GAIN MUSCLE (OPTIONAL)		
Bench Reverse Hyper (p.86)	2	15
GET LEAN (OPTIONAL)		
Pop Squat (p.182)	3	30 sec.

DAY 5

CHEST/BICEPS/TRICEPS

EXERCISE	SETS	REPS/DURATION
SUPERSET		
Dumbbell Incline Bench Press (p.116)	3	10
Spider Curl (p.136)	3	15
SUPERSET		
Bench Dip (p.130)	3	10–12
Dumbbell Incline Flye (p.122)	3	12
SUPERSET		

EXERCISE	SETS	REPS/DURATION
Standing Biceps Curl (p.132)	3	10
Incline Push-Up (p.121)	3	12
GIANT SET		
Decline Push-Up (p.120)	2	AMRAP
Triceps Kickback (p.128)	2	12
Seated Biceps Curl (p.113)	2	12
GAIN MUSCLE (OPTIONAL)		
Dumbbell Squeeze Press (p.119)	2	12
GET LEAN (OPTIONAL)		
Dumbbell Swing (p.180)	5	20 sec.

DAY 6

SHOULDERS

EXERCISE	SETS	REPS/DURATION
Banded Shoulder Press (p.145)	3	8
Lateral Raise (p.152)	3	10
Y-Press (p.145)	3	15
SUPERSET		
Bus Driver (p.156)	3	20 total
Dumbbell Face Pull (p.148)	3	20
SUPERSET		
Dumbbell Press-Out (p.150)	3	15
Reverse Flye (p.154)	3	15
GAIN MUSCLE (OPTIONAL)		
Banded Face Pull (p.149)	2	20
GET LEAN (OPTIONAL)		
Bear Crawl (p.185)	2	30 sec.

ABS CIRCUIT

EXERCISE	SETS	REPS/DURATION
Vacuum (p.161)	4	15–20 sec.
Knee-Up (p.164)	2	25–30
Banded Bicycle (p.167)	2	40 (total)
Reverse Crunch (p.171)	2	20–25

DAY 7 (REST)

CONTINUES...

6-DAY PUSH-PULL-LEGS PROGRAM

By focusing on movements, you're able to effectively train muscle groups that ordinarily work together. For example, when training chest, you'll also hit shoulders and triceps. And by training them together in one day, you'll be able to work all the muscles involved in a specific movement. This gives you two days of training per week for each muscle group, which can lead to greater gains over time. This also gives you more time to recover between workouts.

DAY 1 — PUSH / ABS

EXERCISE	SETS	REPS/DURATION
Decline Push-Up (p.120)	3	AMRAP
Y-Press (p.145)	3	8
SUPERSET		
Lateral Raise (p.152)	3	10
Single Dumbbell Front Raise (p.157)	3	10
SUPERSET		
Dumbbell Incline Flye (p.122)	3	10
Incline Bench Triceps Kickback (p.129)	3	12
SUPERSET		
Dumbbell Squeeze Press (p.119)	3	10
Dumbbell Skullcrusher (p.138)	3	10
GAIN MUSCLE (OPTIONAL)		
Seated Shoulder Press (p.144)	2	10
GET LEAN (OPTIONAL)		
Bear Crawl (p.185)	3	30 sec.

ABS CIRCUIT

EXERCISE	SETS	REPS/DURATION
Lying Leg Raise (p.172)	2	15–20
Dead Bug (p.166)	2	15/side
Flutter Kick (p.166)	2	20/side
Hollow Hold (p.166)	2	30–45 sec.

DAY 2 — PULL

EXERCISE	SETS	REPS/DURATION
Banded Lat Pull-Down (p.92)	3	12
Supine Dumbbell Row (p.102)	3	10
SUPERSET		
Banded Low Row (p.106)	3	12
Banded Biceps Curl (p.134)	3	15
SUPERSET		
Banded Face Pull (p.149)	3	10
High Biceps Curl (p.135)	3	12
SUPERSET		
Single-Arm Dumbbell Row (p.104)	3	8/side
Single-Arm Dumbbell Pull-Over (p.99)	3	8/side
GAIN MUSCLE (OPTIONAL)		
Yates Row (p.100)	2	10
GET LEAN (OPTIONAL)		
Wall Sprint (p.181)	5	20 sec.

DAY 3 — LEGS

EXERCISE	SETS	REPS/DURATION
Goblet Bench Squat (p.63)	3	10
Hip Thrust (p.76)	3	12
SUPERSET		
Dumbbell Deficit Deadlift (p.75)	3	10
Standing Calf Raise (p.88)	3	20
SUPERSET		
Lateral Lunge (p.65)	3	8/side
Offset Bulgarian Split Squat (p.67)	3	8/side
SUPERSET		
Dumbbell Good Morning (p.82)	3	12
Spanish Squat (p.84)	3	15
GAIN MUSCLE (OPTIONAL)		
Bulgarian Split Squat (p.66)	2	10/side
GET LEAN (OPTIONAL)		
Dumbbell Thruster (p.187)	3	12–15

DAY 4

PUSH

EXERCISE	SETS	REPS/DURATION
Seated Shoulder Press (p.144)	3	AMRAP
Banded Lateral Raise (p.153)	3	8
SUPERSET		
Banded Shoulder Press (p.145)	3	8–10
Banded Upright Row (p.147)	3	12
SUPERSET		
Reverse Flye (p.154)	3	15
Triceps Kickback (p.128)	3	12
SUPERSET		
Dumbbell Press-Out (p.150)	3	10
Bench Dip (p.130)	3	8–10
GAIN MUSCLE (OPTIONAL)		
Bus Driver (p.156)	2	20 (total)
GET LEAN (OPTIONAL)		
Incline Mountain Climber (p.186)	5	30 sec.

DAY 5

PULL (BICEPS-FOCUSED) / ABS

EXERCISE	SETS	REPS/DURATION
High-Incline Supine Row (p.103)	3	12
Wide-Grip Pull-Down (p.93)	3	15
SUPERSET		
Dumbbell Pull-Over (p.98)	3	12
Seated Banded Row (p.96)	3	15
SUPERSET		
Bent-Over Row (p.105)	3	8
Standing Biceps Curl (p.132)	3	8–10
SUPERSET		
Single-Arm Side Pull-Down (p.110)	3	10/side
Cross-Body Curl (p.133)	3	8/side
GAIN MUSCLE (OPTIONAL)		
Seated Banded Row (p.96)	1	AMRAP
GET LEAN (OPTIONAL)		
Burpee (p.176)	4	20 sec.

ABS CIRCUIT

EXERCISE	SETS	REPS/DURATION
Vacuum (p.161)	4	10–15 sec.
Banded Crunch (p.162)	4	30
Knee-Up (p.164)	4	20–25
Toe Toucher (p.170)	4	20–25
Alternating Lying Leg Raise (p.173)	4	30 (total)

DAY 6

LEGS

EXERCISE	SETS	REPS/DURATION
Dumbbell Deadlift (p.74)	3	15
Mini-Band Straight-Leg Deadlift (p.73)	3	12
SUPERSET		
Cossack Squat (p.64)	3	8/side
Single-Leg Bench-Assisted Squat (p.60)	3	8/side
SUPERSET		
Banded Pull-Through (p.83)	3	15
Standing Calf Raise (p.88)	3	15
SUPERSET		
Reverse Nordic Curl (p.80)	3	10–12
Sliding Floor Curl (p.78)	3	8–10
GAIN MUSCLE (OPTIONAL)		
Heel-Elevated Hack Squat (p.68)	2	10
GET LEAN (OPTIONAL)		
Dumbbell Swing (p.180)	4	10–12

DAY 7 (REST)

CONTINUES...

6-DAY HIGH-FREQUENCY SPLIT PROGRAM

If you like to train total-body each time you work out, this program is for you. The overall volume for each muscle group is low, which allows for recovery for the next day. Training the muscle each day can cause enough stimulation to encourage muscle growth. Your overall volume for each muscle group will be very similar to the other 6-day programs, but it's more spread out over the 6 days. This program can also be a great way to break through any plateaus as it's a change from traditional bodybuilding splits.

DAY 1

EXERCISE	SETS	REPS/DURATION
Dumbbell Sumo Deadlift (p.75)	3	8
Straight-Leg Deadlift (p.72)	3	8
Offset Bulgarian Split Squat (p.67)	2	8/side
Seated Shoulder Press (p.144)	3	10
Banded Lateral Raise (p.153)	3	12
SUPERSET		
Dumbbell Squeeze Press (p.119)	3	8
Banded Upright Row (p.147)	3	12
Banded High Row (p.94)	2	10 to 12
GAIN MUSCLE (OPTIONAL)		
Single Dumbbell Front Raise (p.157)	2	8/side
GET LEAN (OPTIONAL)		
Dumbbell Thruster (p.187)	3	15

DAY 2

EXERCISE	SETS	REPS/DURATION
Hip Thrust (p.76)	3	12
Banded Reverse Hyper (p.87)	3	15
Goblet Squat (p.62)	2	15
Wide-Grip Pull-Down (p.93)	3	12
High-Incline Bench Press (p.117)	3	12
SUPERSET		
Dumbbell Pull-Over (p.98)	3	10
Dumbbell Incline Flye (p.122)	3	12
SUPERSET		
Plyo Push-Up (p.184)	1	AMRAP
Cross-Body Curl (p.133)	1	AMRAP
GAIN MUSCLE (OPTIONAL)		
Banded Upright Row (p.147)	2	20
GET LEAN (OPTIONAL SUPERSET)		
Dumbbell Swing (p.180)	2	15
Dumbbell Thruster (p.187)	2	15

ABS CIRCUIT (QUICK)

EXERCISE	SETS	REPS/DURATION
X-Plank (p.160)	1	30–35 sec.
Side Plank (p.168)	1	30–35 sec./side
Hollow Hold (p.166)	1	30–35 sec.
Reverse Crunch (p.171)	1	30–35 sec.

EXERCISE	SETS	REPS/DURATION
Quad Step-Up (p.70)	3	12
Spanish Squat (p.84)	2	15
SUPERSET		
Single-Leg Sliding Floor Curl (p.79)	2	8/side
Reverse Nordic Curl (p.80)	2	10–12
SUPERSET		
Dynamic Step-Up (p.183)	3	8/side
B-Stance Hip Thrust (p.77)	3	8/side
SUPERSET		
Reverse Flye (p.154)	2	12
Triceps Kickback (p.128)	2	15
SUPERSET		
Standing Biceps Curl (p.132)	2	10
Bench Dip (p.130)	2	12
GAIN MUSCLE (OPTIONAL)		
Spider Curl (p.136)	2	15
GET LEAN (OPTIONAL)		
Mountain Climber (p.186)	5	30 sec.

EXERCISE	SETS	REPS/DURATION
Hip Thrust (p.76)	3	8
Banded Pull-Through (p.83)	3	15
Single-Leg Bench-Assisted Squat (p.60)	3	8/side
Single-Arm Side Pull-Down (p.110)	3	10/side
SUPERSET		
Bent Over Row (p.105)	3	8/side
Bench Dip (p.130)	3	10–12
Renegade Row (p.108)	2	20 (total)
GAIN MUSCLE (OPTIONAL)		
Supine Dumbbell Row (p.102)	2	10
GET LEAN (OPTIONAL)		
Pop Squat (p.182)	3	20

ABS CIRCUIT

EXERCISE	SETS	REPS/DURATION
Vacuum (p.161)	3	(as long as you can)
X-Plank (p.160)	3	30–45 sec.
High Plank Leg Lift (p.160)	3	18–20/side

EXERCISE	SETS	REPS/DURATION
Vacuum (p.161)	6–7	(as long as you can)
SUPERSET		
Dumbbell Deadlift (p.74)	3	10
Standing Calf Raise (p.88)	3	8
Split Squat	3	8/side
Y-Press (p.145)	3	15
Lateral Raise (p.152)	3	8
SUPERSET		
Dumbbell Press-Out (p.150)	3	8
Wide-Grip Upright Row (p.146)	3	12
GAIN MUSCLE (OPTIONAL)		
Banded Face Pull (p.149)	2	15
GET LEAN (OPTIONAL)		
Shadow Boxing (p.179)	3	20 sec.

EXERCISE	SETS	REPS/DURATION
Dumbbell Swing (p.180)	3	12
SUPERSET		
Incline Push-Up (p.121)	3	12–15
Cross-Body Curl (p.133)	3	10/side
SUPERSET		
Dumbbell Incline Bench Press (p.116)	3	15
Yates Row (p.100)	3	12
SUPERSET		
Dumbbell Incline Flye (p.122)	2	15
Incline Bench Upright Row (p.149)	2	15
SUPERSET		
Banded Cross-Body Chest Press (p.124)	2	10/side
Banded Triceps Push-Down (p.140)	2	12
GAIN MUSCLE (OPTIONAL)		
Dumbbell Pull-Over (p.98)	2	10
GET LEAN (OPTIONAL)		
High Knees (p.178)	5	20 sec.

DAY 7 (REST)

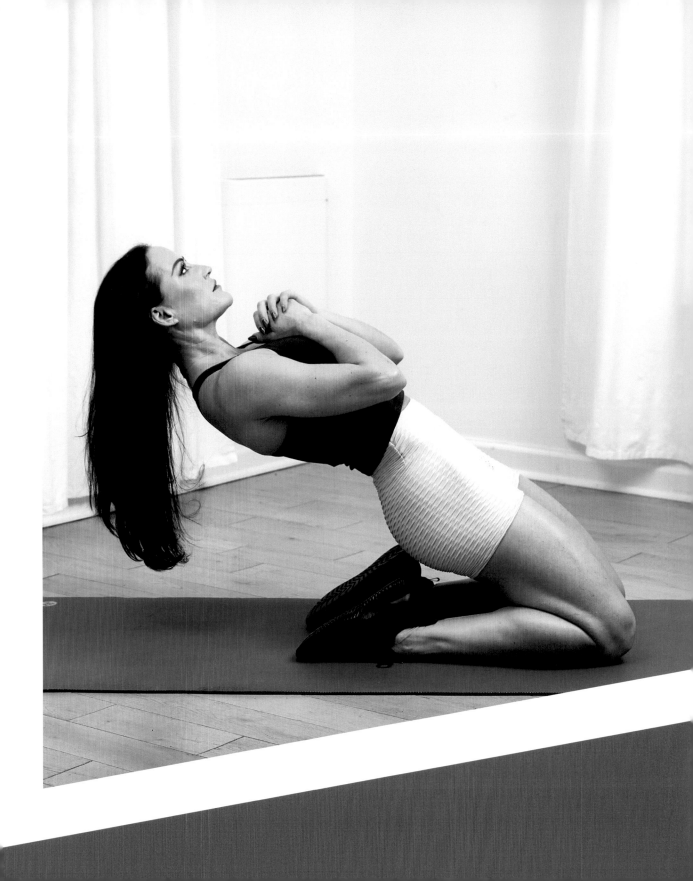

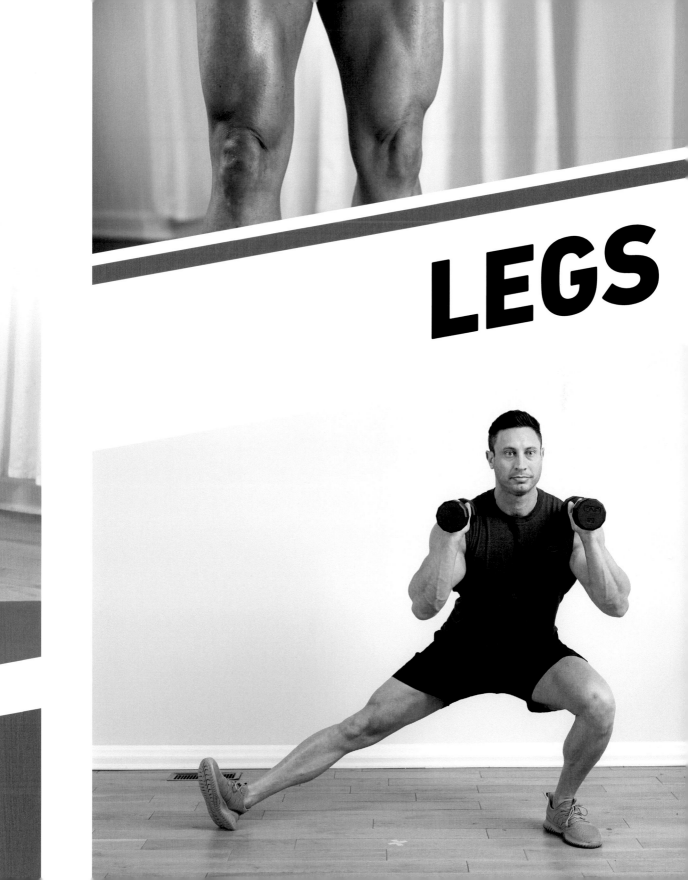

LEGS

TARGETS /// quads, hamstrings, glutes (primary); calves, lower back (secondary)
EQUIPMENT /// bench

SINGLE-LEG BENCH-ASSISTED SQUAT

This squat variation is perfectly suited for home training and can be modified for both beginners and advanced athletes. Single-leg exercises improve overall strength and can help equalize muscle symmetry between the legs.

TRAIN THE RIGHT WAY

DO: Begin with your nondominant leg, and let it dictate the number of reps you do on your dominant leg.

DON'T: Round your back or let your knee cave inward.

[**1**] Stand with your back to the bench and your feet positioned about 12 inches (30.5cm) from the bench. Bring your hands together in front of your chest. Keeping your core tight and back flat, put all of your weight onto one foot, and then lift the other foot off of the floor.

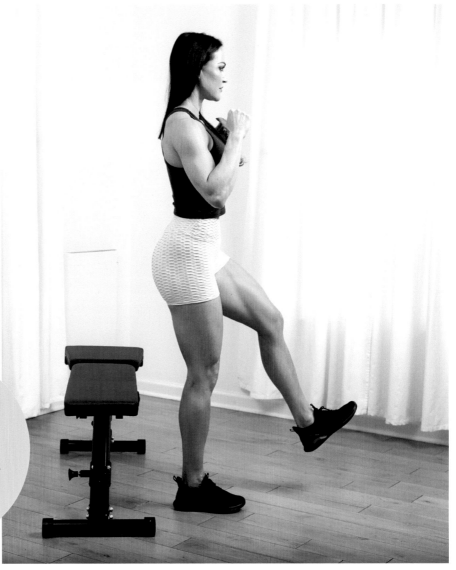

///// **TIP** /////
The knees should always follow the direction of the toes.

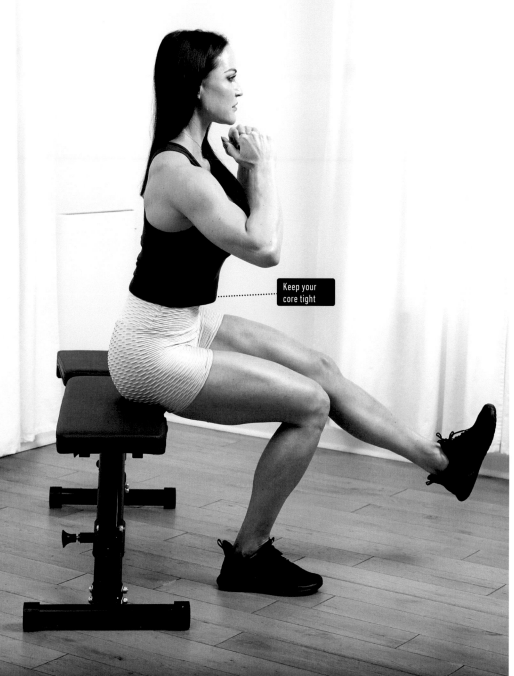

Keep your
core tight

VARIATIONS

B-STANCE (EASIER)
Place the toe of your nonworking leg next to the arch of the foot of your working leg. Focus on using just your working leg while performing the exercise. (The nonworking leg can still be used to help with balance.)

GOBLET SQUAT HOLD (MORE CHALLENGING)
Hold a dumbbell perpendicular to the floor with your palms supporting the top plate. Bring your elbows together underneath the weight, holding them as close to your body as possible. (The top of the dumbbell should almost touch your clavicle.) Perform the exercise as instructed.

[2] With your chest up, slowly bend at the knee and sit back onto the bench, pause momentarily, and then push your weight through your heel as you drive your body back up to the starting point, inhaling as you ascend. Repeat the same number of reps on the opposite leg.

TARGETS /// **quads, glutes (primary); upper back, core (secondary)**
EQUIPMENT /// **dumbbell**

GOBLET SQUAT

This squat variation promotes proper form, which makes it a staple exercise whether you're a beginner or an advanced athlete. The goblet squat has similar benefits to the barbell squat, but it creates much less stress on the back. And since you're holding the weight, your entire body will get a workout, including your hands as they grip the dumbbell.

TRAIN THE RIGHT WAY

DO: Keep your elbows positioned underneath the dumbbell, and keep the dumbbell close to your body.

DON'T: Round your back as this can cause pain and cause you to lose balance.

[1] Hold a dumbbell perpendicular to the ground with your palms positioned underneath the top plate. Bring your elbows in, holding them as close to your body as possible. Stand with your feet positioned slightly wider than your shoulders.

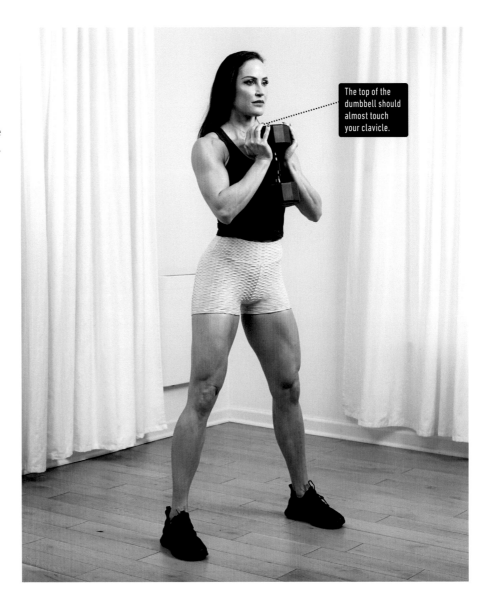

The top of the dumbbell should almost touch your clavicle.

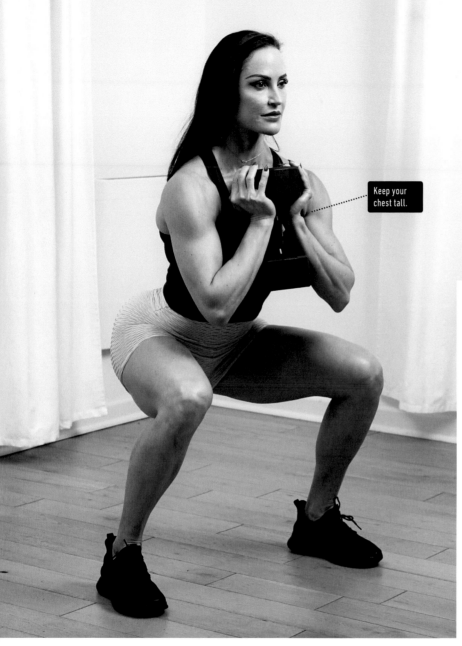

Keep your chest tall.

TIP
The knees should always follow the direction of the toes.

VARIATIONS

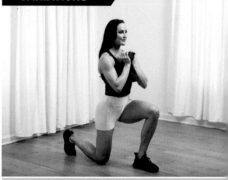

GOBLET SKATER SQUAT (MORE CHALLENGING) Hold a light dumbbell with your palms positioned underneath the top plate. Stand with your feet together. Slowly step one leg back into a reverse lunge. (As you step back, try to use only your front leg to lower yourself down.) Push yourself back up, and then repeat on the opposite side.

GOBLET BENCH SQUAT (EASIER) Stand with your back to a bench. Hold the dumbbell with your palms positioned underneath the top plate. Slowly sit back onto the bench, pause briefly, and then drive yourself back up to the starting position. (This variation improves power and reinforces mind-muscle connection.)

[2] Using the dumbbell to counterbalance your body as you lower yourself, slowly bend your knees and push your hips back as you sit back until your upper legs are parallel to the floor, and then push your weight through your heels to slowly push yourself back up to the starting position.

TARGETS /// **quads, hamstrings, glutes (primary); calves, core (secondary)**
EQUIPMENT /// **dumbbells**

COSSACK SQUAT

This squat variation will not only sculpt the legs but also improve lower body flexibility and mobility. Since this squat variation is a hybrid between a single-leg and a bilateral exercise, you'll reap the benefits of single-leg training, including improved symmetry from the right to left side and improved strength, and you'll also enjoy the stability benefits of a bilateral exercise.

TRAIN THE RIGHT WAY

DO: Start with just your bodyweight and try to focus on using proper form before adding weight.

DON'T: Allow the working knee to cave inward at any time as this can cause pain or injury.

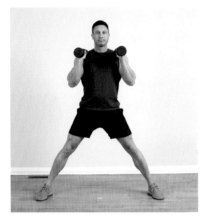

[**1**] Place the dumbbells on the fronts of your shoulders with your elbows positioned directly beneath the dumbbells. Stand with your feet positioned about twice the width of your shoulders, with your toes pointing slightly outward.

[**2**] Slowly bend one leg, dropping your hips down directly over the bending leg. Extend your nonworking leg straight while slowly bringing your nonworking toe off the floor until the working upper leg reaches parallel to the floor. Keep your chest up and your back flat as you descend. Pause momentarily in this position. (It should look like a lateral lunge.)

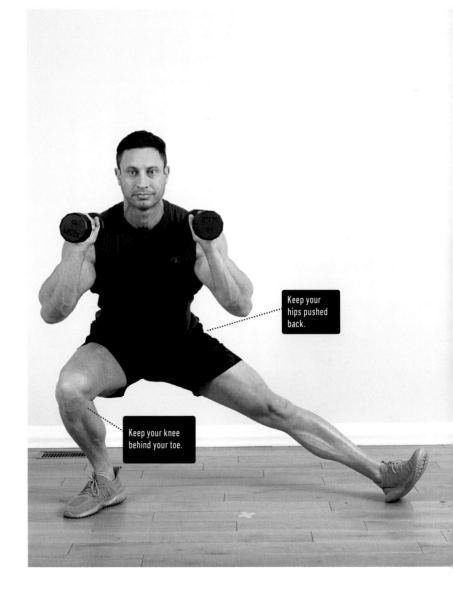

Keep your hips pushed back.

Keep your knee behind your toe.

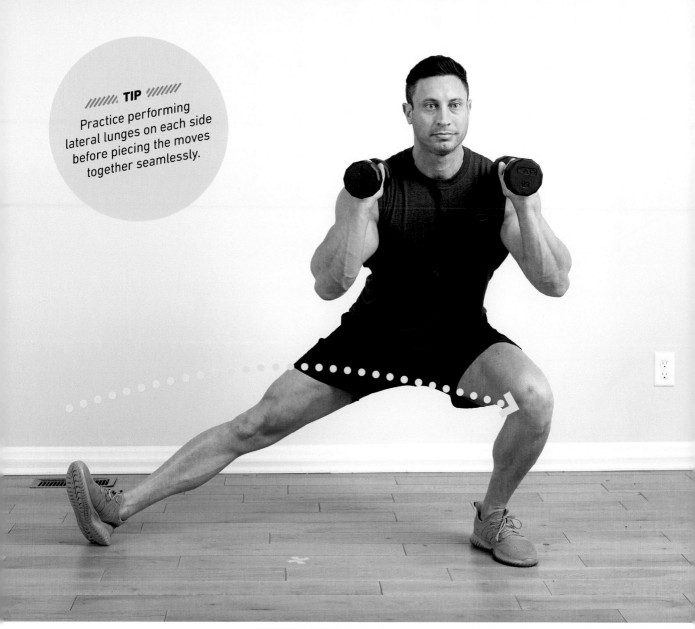

TIP
Practice performing lateral lunges on each side before piecing the moves together seamlessly.

[**3**] In one motion, slowly rise up to the starting position and then down to the opposite leg. Slowly alternate the motion back and forth in a continuous fashion, maintaining constant tension throughout the exercise and pausing briefly at the bottom of the movement on each side.

VARIATIONS

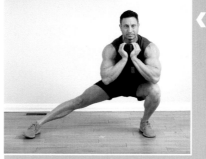

LATERAL LUNGE (EASIER) Perform all reps on one side before shifting to the opposite side. (These can be done with just bodyweight or while holding a dumbbell.)

LOW COSSACK SQUAT (MORE CHALLENGING) Begin the exercise as instructed, but instead of rising all the way back up to the starting position, only rise up enough to be able to switch sides.

TARGETS /// **glutes, hamstrings, quads (primary); calves, core (secondary)**
EQUIPMENT /// **bench, dumbbells**

BULGARIAN SPLIT SQUAT

This squat variation trains one leg at a time and allows you to train your legs harder but without going as heavy as you would for a traditional squat. The result is muscle gain, increased power, and improved balance. This movement can also balance out asymmetries and improve core strength.

TRAIN THE RIGHT WAY

DO: Focus on pushing with your front leg rather than pulling with the rear leg.

DON'T: Lean forward with your upper body.

[**1**] Face away from the bench. Hold the dumbbells at your sides with your arms extended downward. Extend one leg backward until your toe is resting on the bench. (Your stance should be staggered, and you should be far enough from the bench that your rear lower leg is parallel to the floor.)

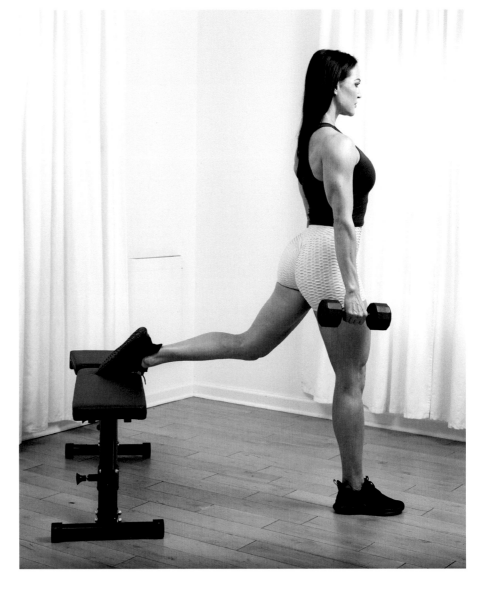

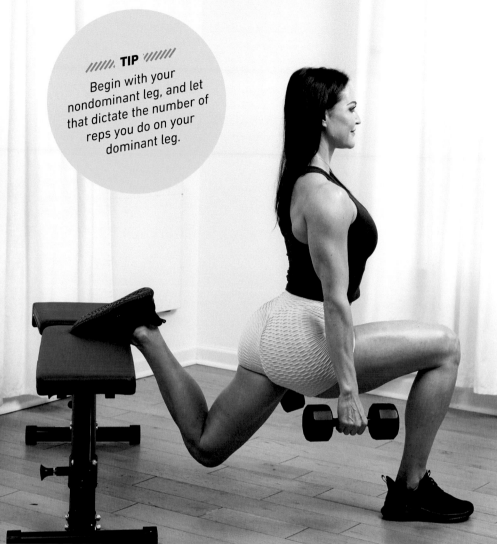

[2] Lower your body until your lead upper leg is parallel to the floor, keeping your body upright with your chest tall. Keep your weight primarily through your front foot, and push your body back up to the starting position. (Be sure to keep your upper body balanced between the lead and trail leg throughout the range of motion.)

///// **TIP** /////
Begin with your nondominant leg, and let that dictate the number of reps you do on your dominant leg.

VARIATIONS

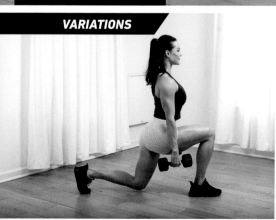

SPLIT SQUAT (EASIER)
This variation does not use a bench. Stand in a lunge position and lower your body until your front upper leg reaches parallel. Switch legs and repeat on the opposite side to complete the set. (This variation works well for beginners or for those who have issues with balance.)

OFFSET BULGARIAN SPLIT SQUAT (MORE CHALLENGING) Hold a dumbbell in the opposite hand of the working leg. (This variation targets the core and glutes more effectively.)

TARGETS /// **quads, hamstrings, glutes (primary); calves (secondary)**
EQUIPMENT /// **dumbbells, weight plates or sturdy old books**

HEEL-ELEVATED HACK SQUAT

The heel-elevated hack squat changes the exercise angle and weight distribution of a traditional squat to better target specific muscle groups. It requires a bit of resourcefulness in order to elevate your heels, but if you want to build a strong quad sweep, this exercise should be included in your regular routine.

TRAIN THE RIGHT WAY

DO: Push your weight through your toes to accentuate quad muscle recruitment.

DON'T: Hunch forward or allow your back to round.

[1] Place two small weight plates or books on the floor, spaced shoulder width apart. Stand with your heels on the plates and hold the dumbbells at your sides and slightly behind you.

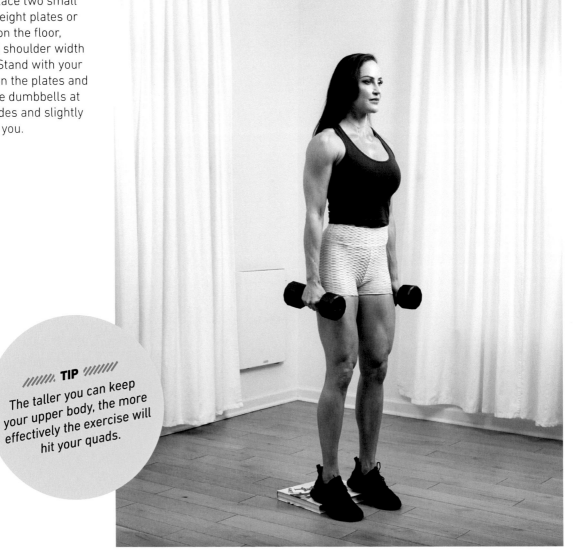

////// **TIP** //////
The taller you can keep your upper body, the more effectively the exercise will hit your quads.

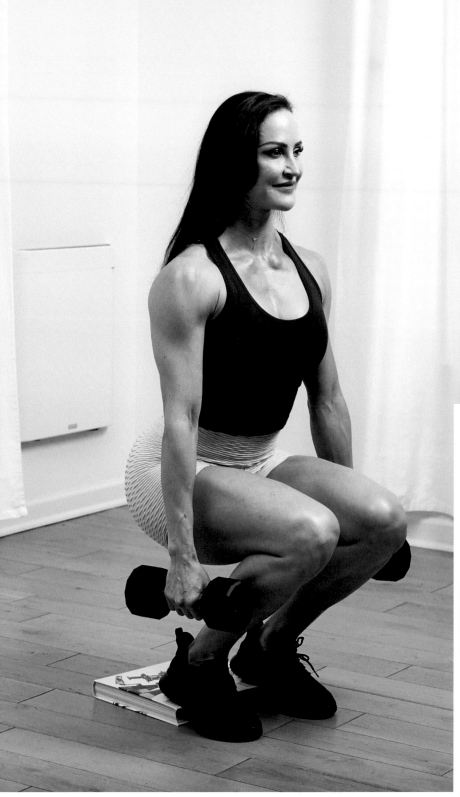

[2] Keeping your upper body tall, push your weight through your toes as you lower your hips to the floor. Pause momentarily when your upper legs reach parallel or just below. Focusing on using just your quads, push through your toes to push yourself back up to the starting position.

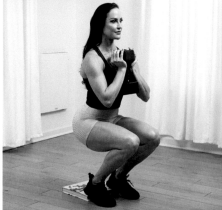

HEEL-ELEVATED GOBLET SQUAT Grasp the end of a dumbbell with your palms positioned underneath the top plate and directly over your elbows. Perform the exercise as instructed. (This variation can allow for a greater range of motion than a normal goblet squat.)

TARGETS /// **quads (primary); hamstrings, glutes, calves (secondary)**
EQUIPMENT /// **bench**

QUAD STEP-UP

You can build impressive quads with this squat alternative. The focus should be on slowing down the exercise tempo, using only your lead leg to pull your body up and using your body as resistance. As an added benefit, you'll improve your balance and body awareness.

TRAIN THE RIGHT WAY

DO: Pay attention to form, and keep your knee in-line with your toe. Pull your body up with your lead leg.

DON'T: Push off with your trail leg.

[1] Stand facing a flat bench. Place one foot on top of the bench with the other foot flat on the floor.

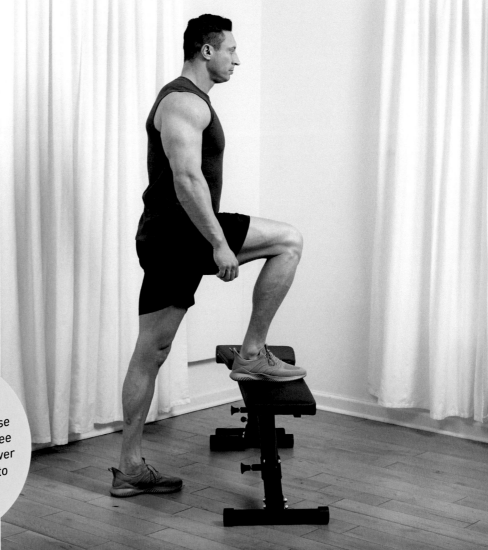

///// **TIP** /////
Keep the trail foot dorsiflexed to limit its use by keeping the back knee slightly bent as you lower yourself back down to the starting point.

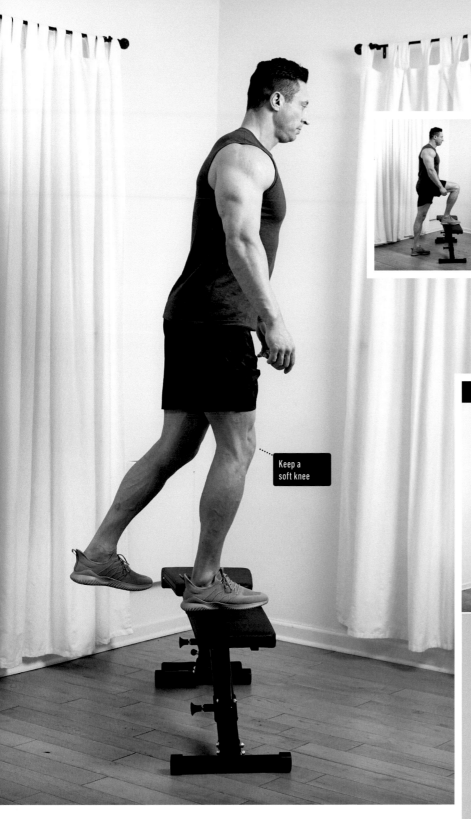

[2] Pull your body up to a standing position on top of the bench.

[3] Using the same leg, slowly step down from the bench. Repeat all reps on one leg before switching to the opposite leg.

Keep a soft knee

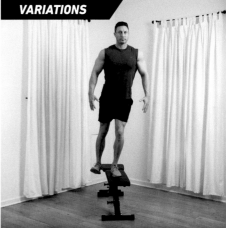

VARIATIONS

LATERAL STEP-UP (MORE CHALLENGING) Stand next to the bench, and place your foot on top of the bench. Slowly pull yourself up to a standing position, and then lower yourself back down. (This variation targets the glutes more effectively.)

OFFSET STEP-UP (MORE CHALLENGING) Hold a dumbbell in the hand opposite your working leg. This will challenge core stability and work the abs.

TARGETS /// **hamstrings (primary); glutes, lower back (secondary)**
EQUIPMENT /// **dumbbells**

STRAIGHT-LEG DEADLIFT

This deadlift variation not only will develop strong and shapely hamstrings and glutes but can also improve flexibility and core strength. A strong posterior chain can result in more explosiveness and the ability to excel in sports.

TRAIN THE RIGHT WAY

DO: Concentrate on pushing your hips back as you lower the dumbbells.

DON'T: Round your lower back or upper back at all during the exercise.

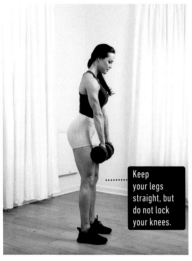

Keep your legs straight, but do not lock your knees.

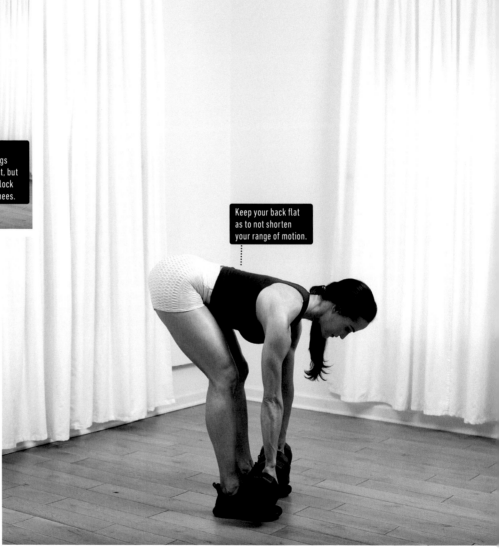

Keep your back flat as to not shorten your range of motion.

[1] Stand tall with your feet shoulder width apart. Hold dumbbells in each hand, keeping them just in front of your legs.

[2] With a tight core and a flat back, slowly lower the dumbbells down to the floor, stopping the descent just before your lower back rounds. (Think about using your hips as a hinge and pushing your hips back as you lower the dumbbells.)

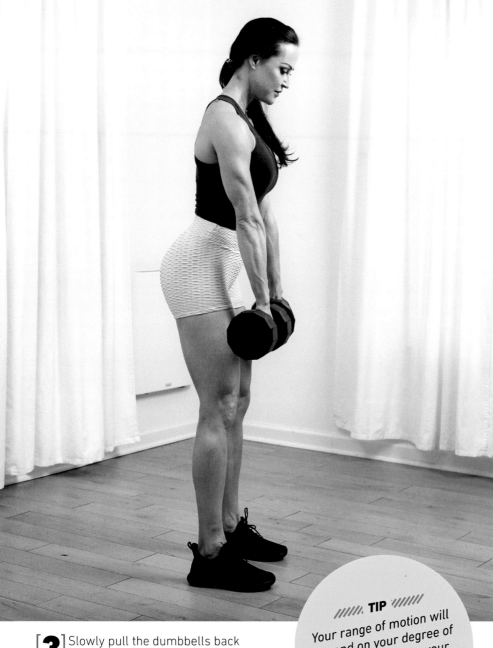

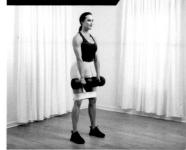

VARIATIONS

🔺 **MINI-BAND STRAIGHT-LEG DEADLIFT (MORE CHALLENGING)**
Place a mini band around your legs and just below the knees. As you perform the exercise, push your knees out against the band. This will increase glute activity.

B-STANCE STRAIGHT-LEG DEADLIFT (MORE CHALLENGING) Using lighter weights, place one foot flat on the floor and the toe of your other foot next to the arch of your flat foot. Perform the exercise as instructed, performing all reps on one leg before switching to the other leg.

ROMANIAN DEADLIFT (RDL) Perform the exercise as instructed, except bend your knees slightly and shorten the range of motion to stop at about shin height before pulling the dumbbells back to the starting point.

[**3**] Slowly pull the dumbbells back up to the starting position, keeping them close to the front of your legs as you rise and pushing your weight through your heels to maintain a neutral spine.

///// **TIP** /////
Your range of motion will depend on your degree of flexibility and also your lower back flatness during the rep.

TARGETS /// **hamstrings, glutes, back (primary); shoulders, calves (secondary)**
EQUIPMENT /// **dumbbell**

DUMBBELL DEADLIFT

A true total body movement, the dumbbell deadlift will increase your overall strength and add muscle to your frame. With the weight distribution in-line with your body, it's a safer lift than the traditional barbell deadlift. And since it's a total body movement, you'll enjoy an increased calorie burn, and you'll be able to get a better workout in a shorter time.

TRAIN THE RIGHT WAY

DO: Limit your range of motion to ensure your back stays flat and your spine stays neutral.

DON'T: Look up as you pull the dumbbell to mid rep.

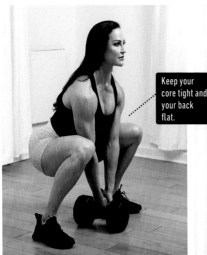

Keep your core tight and your back flat.

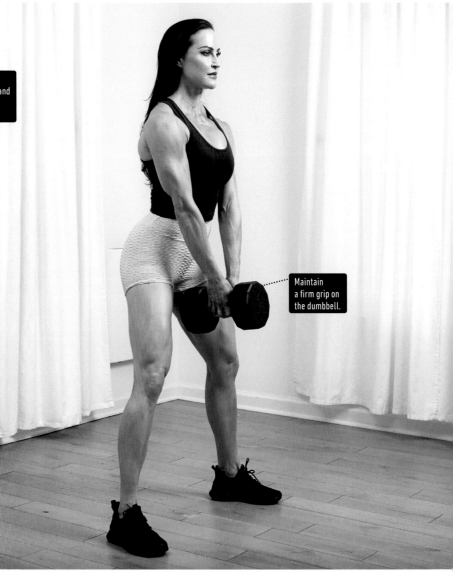

Maintain a firm grip on the dumbbell.

[**1**] Stand with your feet positioned about one and a half times shoulder width. Place a dumbbell on the floor between your feet with the handle parallel to your feet. Lower down slowly, pushing your hips back while keeping your upper body tall. Interlock your fingers underneath the handle.

[**2**] Slowly pull the dumbbell upward, using your legs, glutes, and upper back to lift. (Think about extending your legs first and then opening your hips fully.) Pause momentarily as you stand fully upright.

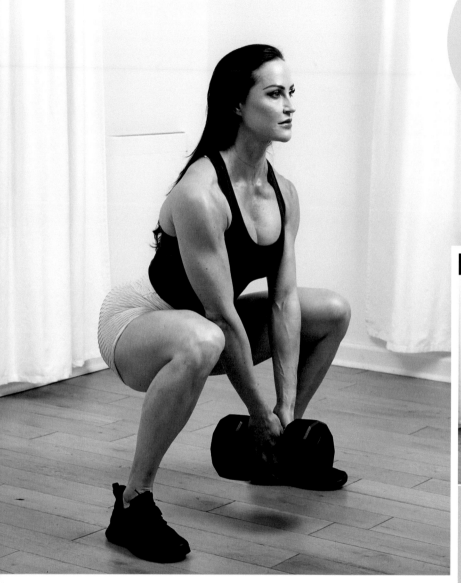

///// TIP /////

If your hips are highly flexible, you can stand on a platform to get full range of motion.

VARIATIONS

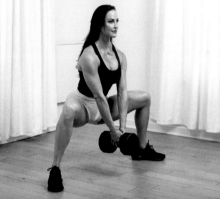

DUMBBELL SUMO DEADLIFT (MORE CHALLENGING) Stand with your feet positioned about double shoulder width apart. Point your toes and knees slightly outward. (This variation hits the adductors more.)

DUMBBELL DEFICIT DEADLIFT (MORE CHALLENGING) Stand on two sturdy books, and perform the exercise as instructed. (This variation extends the range of motion of the exercise and can target the glutes more.)

[3] Slowly lower back down into the starting position, but don't let the dumbbell rest on the floor.

TARGETS /// **glutes, hamstrings (primary); quads, lower back (secondary)**
EQUIPMENT /// **bench, dumbbell**

HIP THRUST

Very few exercises target just the glutes like the hip thrust. It can build strength for other lifts and create power that translates well to sports. In addition to performance improvements, this hip-extension movement creates full and round glutes, which can make the waist appear smaller and lend strong curves to the lower body.

TRAIN THE RIGHT WAY

DO: Focus on keeping an anterior tilt in the pelvis. (This will engage the glutes better.)

DON'T: Place your feet too far out in front of you as this will work the hamstrings.

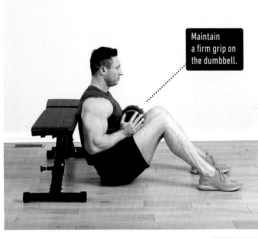

Maintain a firm grip on the dumbbell.

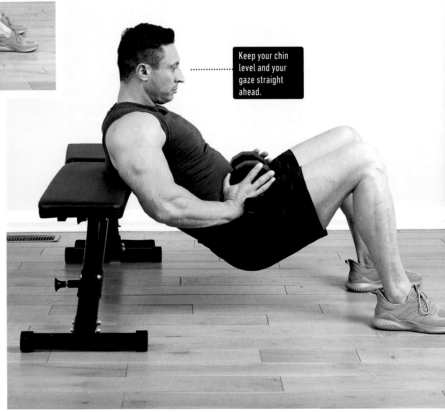

Keep your chin level and your gaze straight ahead.

[1] Sit on the floor with your back to the long side of a flat bench. Pull your knees close to your chest, with your feet flat on the floor. Position your upper back against the bench pad. Gently place a dumbbell over your hips.

[2] Rise into the starting position by lifting your hips off the floor.

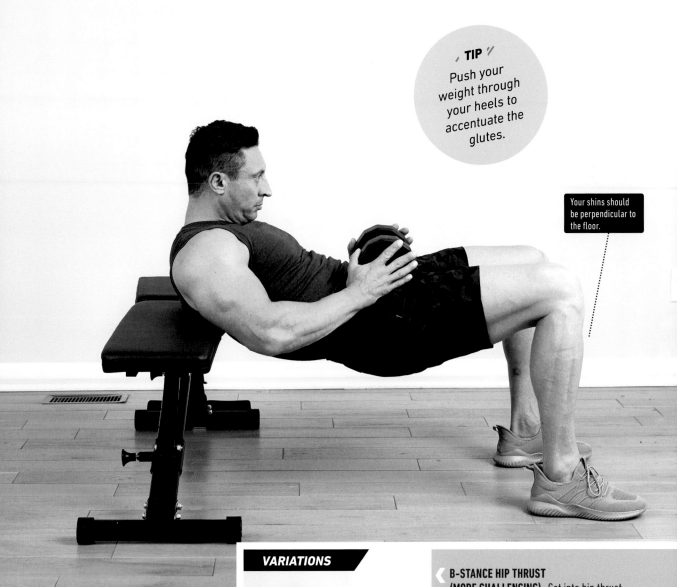

⟋ TIP ⟍
Push your weight through your heels to accentuate the glutes.

Your shins should be perpendicular to the floor.

[**3**] Push your hips upward until you reach a full hip extension, keeping your chin tucked to your chest, and then slowly lower your hips back down to the starting position.

VARIATIONS

‹ B-STANCE HIP THRUST (MORE CHALLENGING) Get into hip thrust position. Lift one heel off the floor, and place your toe next to the arch of the foot that's on the ground. Perform the exercise as instructed, using just the working leg (flat foot) to push. Switch sides and repeat.

MINI-BAND HIP THRUST (MORE CHALLENGING) Place a resistance band around your legs and just below your knees. Perform the exercise as instructed, but try to push against the resistance band as you perform the exercise. (This variation works the abductors along with the glutes.)

TARGETS /// **hamstrings (primary); calves, glutes, core (secondary)**
EQUIPMENT /// **yoga mat, towel or paper plates**

SLIDING FLOOR CURL

This bodyweight exercise is the perfect substitute for the leg-curl machine. Since you're using just your body weight, you can increase or reduce the difficulty by adjusting your tempo and level of muscle contraction. Strong hamstrings directly contribute to increased power and can also decrease injury risk.

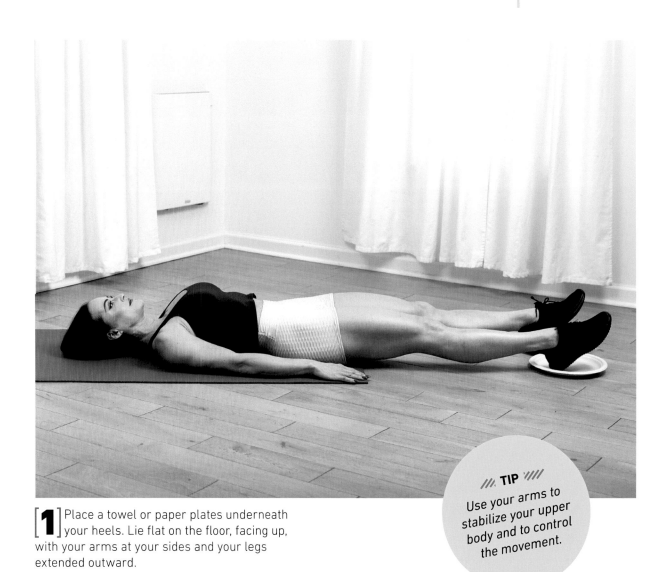

[**1**] Place a towel or paper plates underneath your heels. Lie flat on the floor, facing up, with your arms at your sides and your legs extended outward.

/// TIP ///
Use your arms to stabilize your upper body and to control the movement.

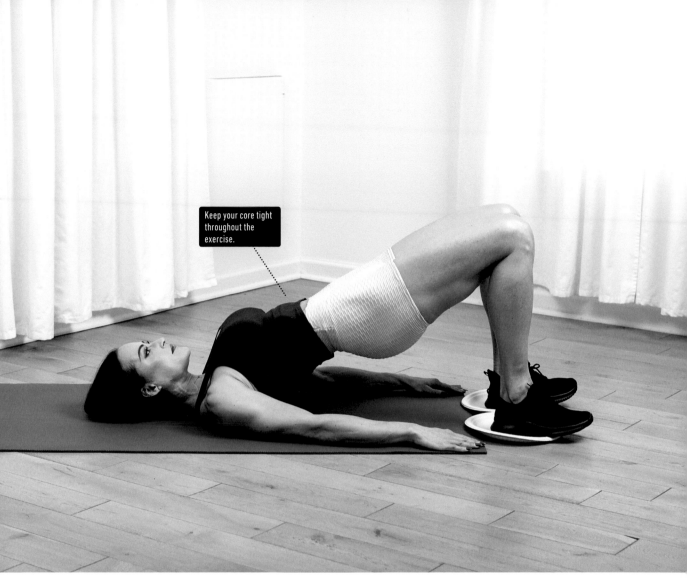

Keep your core tight throughout the exercise.

[2] Slowly pull your heels in toward your glutes as you lift your hips off the floor, focusing on using just your hamstrings to move your body. Keep your core tight, and keep your hips and shoulders in a straight line. Continue pulling with your hamstrings until your shins are perpendicular to the floor (as your heels get closer to your glutes, your hips should continue to rise), pause momentarily, and then slowly push your heels back out, extending your legs down to the starting point.

VARIATIONS

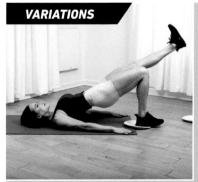

SINGLE-LEG SLIDING FLOOR CURL (MORE CHALLENGING) Extend one leg off the floor, and perform the exercise using just the working leg. Repeat on the opposite side.

SINGLE-LEG NEGATIVE SLIDING FLOOR CURL (MORE CHALLENGING) Begin the exercise as instructed. Once your shins reach perpendicular to the floor, slowly lift one leg off the floor and perform the negative portion of the rep using just the working leg. Repeat the beginning steps and alternate the negatives on each side.

TARGETS /// **quads, hip flexors (primary); core (secondary)**
EQUIPMENT /// **yoga mat**

REVERSE NORDIC CURL

It can be incredibly difficult to target just the quads at home, but with the reverse Nordic curl, you can successfully train just the quads and also control the level of difficulty. You only need a yoga mat and your body weight to do this exercise effectively. In addition to building muscle, reverse Nordic curls can build strength and help alleviate back pain by strengthening the hip flexors and core.

TRAIN THE RIGHT WAY

DO: Focus on the negative, or lowering, portion of the movement.

DON'T: Break at the hips as this can remove tension from the quads.

[1] Get into a tall kneeling position on a yoga mat with your knees positioned shoulder width apart, your toes pointed away from you, and the tops of your feet flat on the mat. Cross your arms in front of your body at chest level.

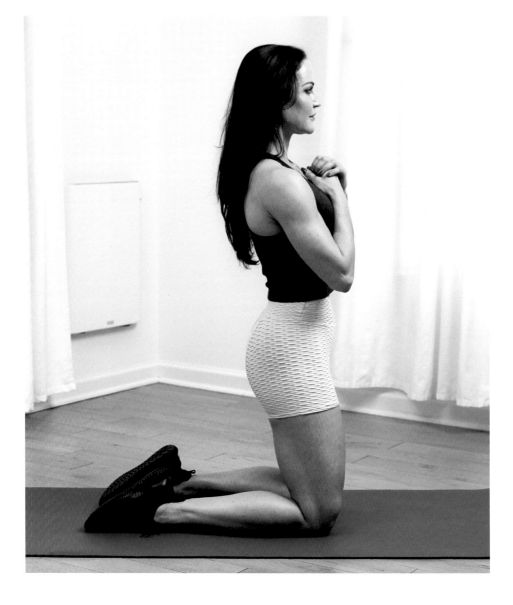

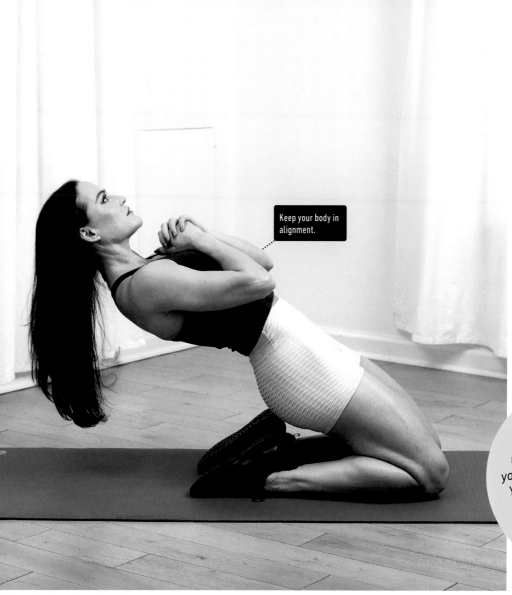

Keep your body in alignment.

[2] Keeping your upper body stiff and your core tight, slowly lower your body back toward your lower legs, focusing on your knees as the hinge-points and using your quads to control the movement. Pause for a moment at the lowest comfortable point, and then use your quads to pull yourself back up to the starting position.

/// **TIP** ///
Try to limit the range of motion when you're just getting started. You can lower your body more and more as you become more accustomed to the exercise.

VARIATIONS

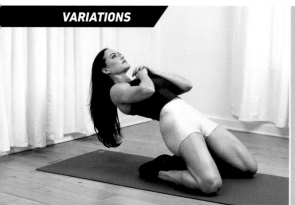

WIDE-STANCE REVERSE NORDIC CURL (MORE CHALLENGING) When getting into position, take a wider stance with your knees. (This advanced variation allows you to drop your upper body all the way to the mat without your lower legs getting in the way.)

BAND-ASSISTED REVERSE NORDIC CURL (EASIER) Place a strong band around a sturdy object that is positioned at about chin height when you're in a tall kneeling position. Face the anchor point and place the band around your lower back. (The band will act as a spotter, making the exercise easier to perform.)

TARGETS /// **hamstrings, glutes, lower back (primary); core (secondary)**
EQUIPMENT /// **dumbbell**

DUMBBELL GOOD MORNING

Good mornings are one of the most effective exercises for working the posterior chain and can help improve strength, power, and aesthetic gains. When training from home, many tend to skip this exercise as it's typically done with a barbell, but this variation allows you to get the same benefits while just using a dumbbell. Start with lighter weight, and go up once you become proficient.

[1] Grasp a dumbbell by placing one hand on each end. Stand with your feet shoulder width apart, and then place a slight bend in your knees. Slowly press the dumbbell overhead, and then lower it behind your head until the dumbbell is resting comfortably on your traps.

Maintain a firm grip on the dumbbell.

Your elbows should be aligned with your hands.

///// **TIP** /////
Keep your spine neutral. If you look up or forward, there's a higher chance of arching your back, which can lead to injury.

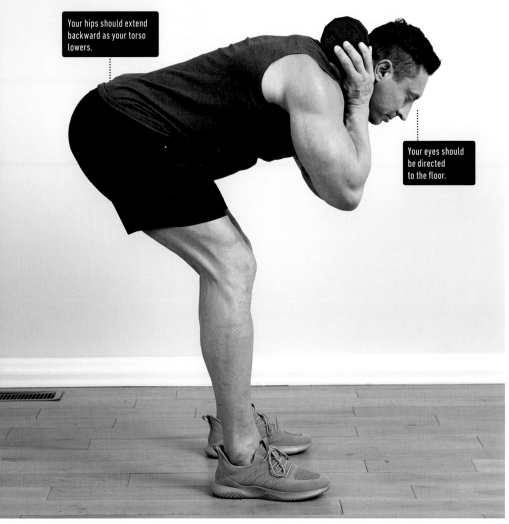

Your hips should extend backward as your torso lowers.

Your eyes should be directed to the floor.

[2] With your head neutral and your back flat, hinge at your hips to lower your upper body down toward the floor. Pause slightly when your upper body is just above parallel or just before your back begins to round, and then engage your hamstrings, glutes, and lower back to raise your body back to the starting position.

VARIATIONS

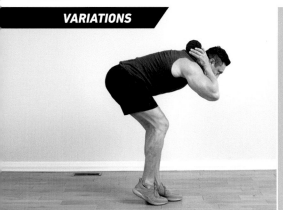

B-STANCE GOOD MORNING (MORE CHALLENGING) Place all of your weight on one leg, and then place the toe of the nonworking leg next to the arch of the foot of the working leg. Perform the exercise, one leg at a time, using the nonworking side to help with balance. (This variation is more advanced and can improve balance and muscle symmetry.)

BANDED PULL-THROUGH Attach a resistance band to a sturdy object at around ankle height. Stand facing away from the band, straddle it, and hold the band with an overhand grip. With your knees slightly bent, hinge your hips as you slowly lower your upper body down toward the floor. (Keep your arms straight, and use them only to stabilize the band.) The movement should be the same as the traditional dumbbell good morning, but the band provides constant tension and can be a safer alternative for those with back issues.

TARGETS /// **quads, hamstrings, glutes (primary); calves, core (secondary)**
EQUIPMENT /// **resistance band**

SPANISH SQUAT

Hit your quads while simultaneously improving knee health with this deceptively difficult squat variation. The Spanish squat can be scaled back to help beginners with form, or weight can be added to make it a staple in an advanced routine. If you miss your local gym's leg-extension machine, this exercise will provide the perfect substitute.

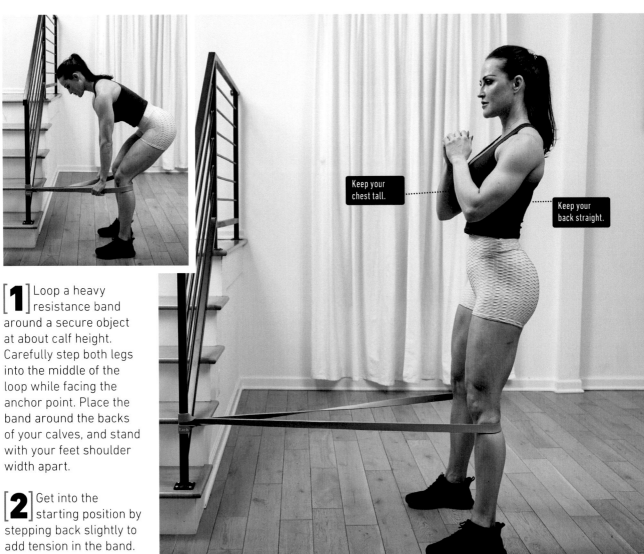

Keep your chest tall.

Keep your back straight.

[**1**] Loop a heavy resistance band around a secure object at about calf height. Carefully step both legs into the middle of the loop while facing the anchor point. Place the band around the backs of your calves, and stand with your feet shoulder width apart.

[**2**] Get into the starting position by stepping back slightly to add tension in the band. Clasp your hands in front of your chest.

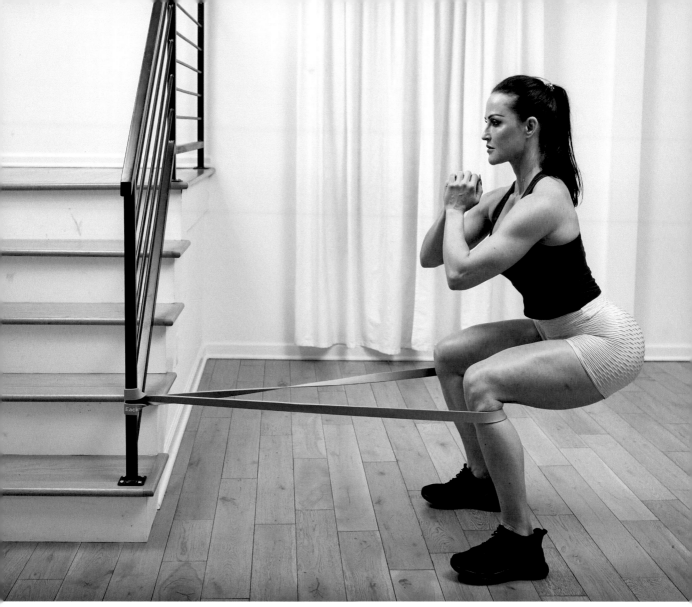

[3] Slowly sit back until your upper leg reaches parallel to the floor, pause momentarily, and then drive your body back up to the starting position. (As you come up, consciously push your knees back against the band and think about contracting your quads.)

VARIATIONS

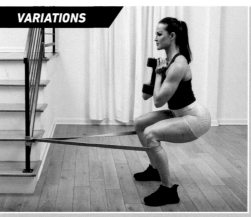

❮ **GOBLET SPANISH SQUAT (MORE CHALLENGING)** Hold a dumbbell perpendicular to the floor with your palms placed underneath the top plate. Bring your elbows directly under the weight and hold them as close together as possible. (The top of the dumbbell should almost touch the clavicle.) Perform the exercise as instructed.

TARGETS /// **hamstrings, glutes (primary); lower back (secondary)**
EQUIPMENT /// **bench**

BENCH REVERSE HYPER

This exercise uses your body weight to strengthen your posterior chain. It's highly effective at targeting the glutes, hamstrings, and lower back. It can also improve hip-extension power and range of motion. And it's easier on the back than traditional weight-loaded exercises. As your strength improves, the bench reverse hyper can be scaled to continue providing a challenge.

TRAIN THE RIGHT WAY

DO: Keep your core engaged throughout the exercise.

DON'T: Lift your legs above parallel with your body as this can put unnecessary pressure on your lower back.

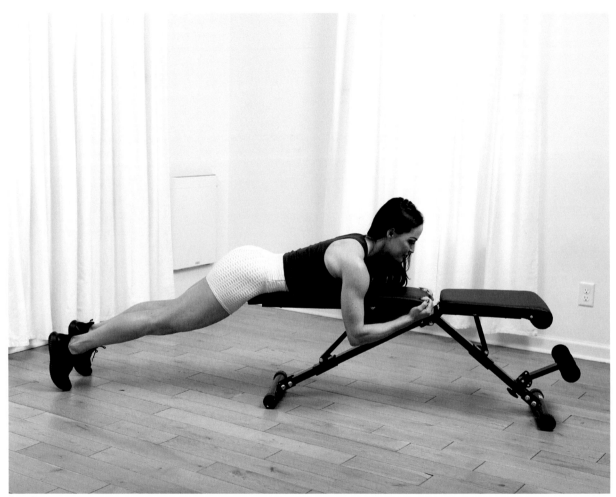

[1] Lie stomach down on a flat bench with your legs hanging off one end of the bench and your toes touching the floor. (Your hip bones should be aligned with the end of the bench, and your toes should be touching the floor.) Grasp the sides of the bench.

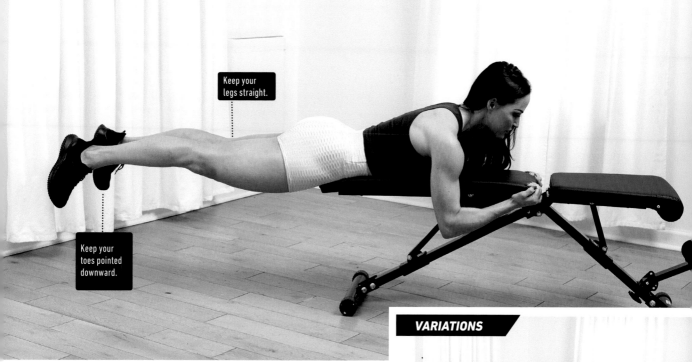

Keep your legs straight.

Keep your toes pointed downward.

[2] Brace your core, push your hips into the bench, and engage your glutes and hamstrings as you lift both legs off the floor simultaneously. Pause briefly when your legs form a straight line with the rest of your body, squeezing your glutes and hamstrings.

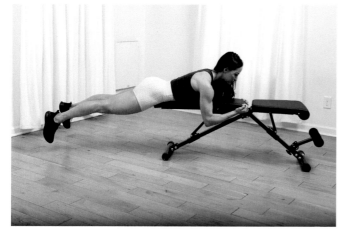

[3] Slowly lower your legs back down until your toes barely touch the floor. Repeat.

VARIATIONS

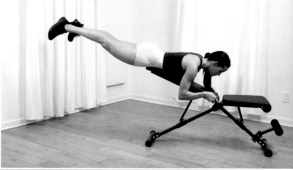

▲ **INCLINE BENCH REVERSE HYPER (MORE CHALLENGING)** If you have an adjustable bench, set it to either 45 or 60 degrees. Lie stomach down on the bench with your hips aligned with the top of the bench. Perform the exercise as instructed. (This variation gives you greater range of motion and increases difficulty.)

BANDED REVERSE HYPER (MORE CHALLENGING) Place a mini band just above your knees, and perform the exercise on a flat or incline bench. As you lift your legs, push against the band to engage the glutes and abductors and make the exercise more challenging.

TARGETS /// **calves**
EQUIPMENT /// **dumbbells**

STANDING CALF RAISE

Calves require both standing and seated exercises to develop the muscles to their full potential. Your calves get considerable stimulation just from walking around during day-to-day activities, so it's important to focus on the lifting cues and ensure you get a good contraction with each rep to work the calves properly.

TRAIN THE RIGHT WAY

DO: Keep your core tight throughout the exercise, and keep the rest of your body still.

DON'T: Use momentum or swing the dumbbells as this can throw you off-balance.

[**1**] Stand with your feet positioned shoulder width apart and flat on the ground so your weight is evenly distributed. Grasp dumbbells in each hand, and place them at your sides.

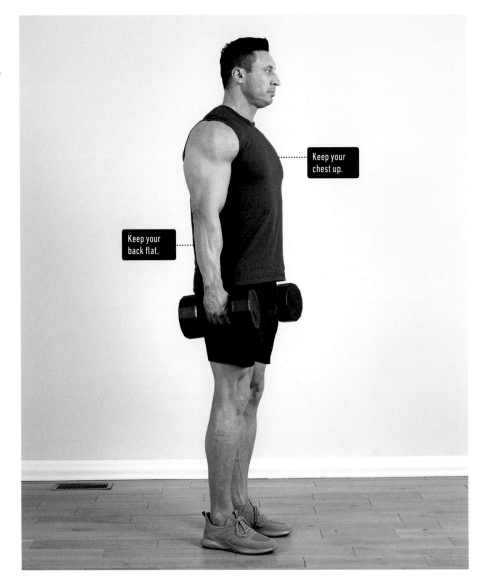

Keep your chest up.

Keep your back flat.

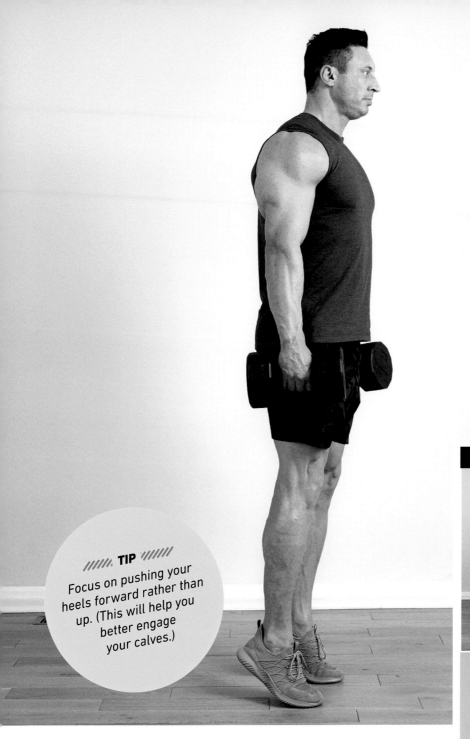

TIP

Focus on pushing your heels forward rather than up. (This will help you better engage your calves.)

[**2**] Slowly shift your weight to your toes, lift your heels off the floor, and squeeze your calves as you rise to the balls of your feet. Pause momentarily, and then slowly lower your heels back down to the starting position.

VARIATIONS

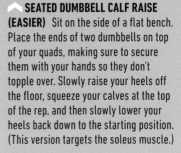

SEATED DUMBBELL CALF RAISE (EASIER) Sit on the side of a flat bench. Place the ends of two dumbbells on top of your quads, making sure to secure them with your hands so they don't topple over. Slowly raise your heels off the floor, squeeze your calves at the top of the rep, and then slowly lower your heels back down to the starting position. (This version targets the soleus muscle.)

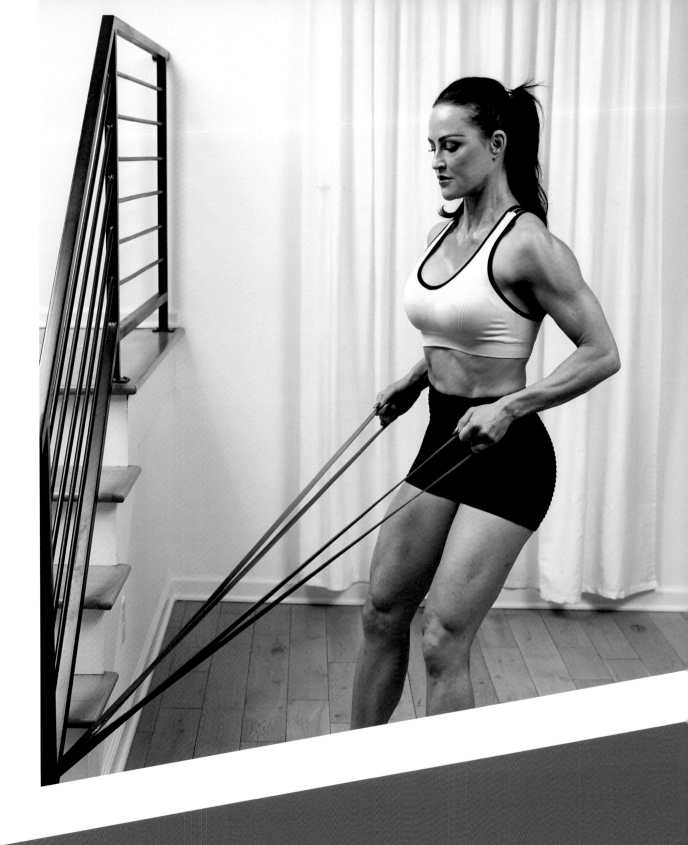

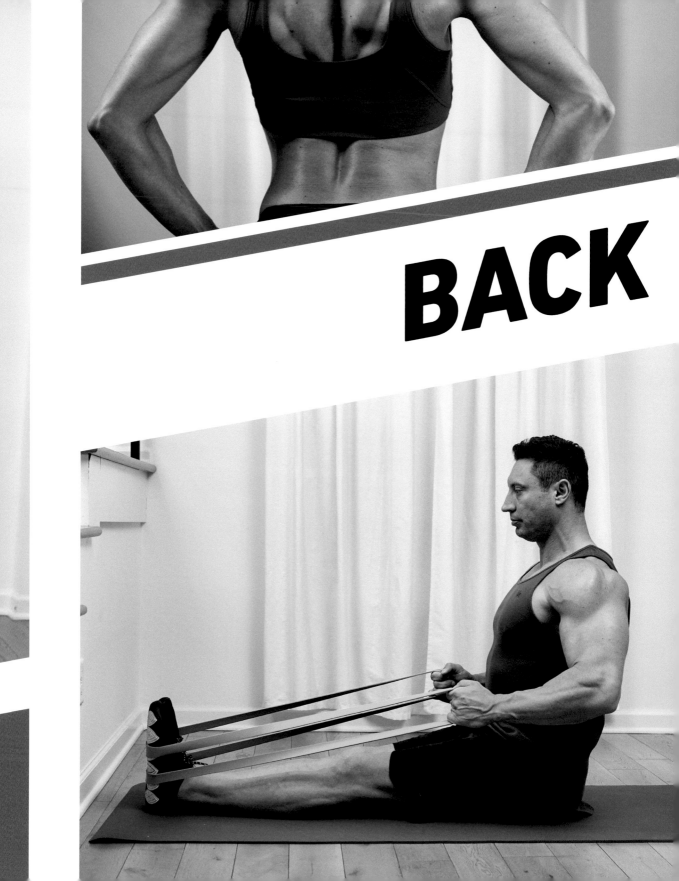

BACK

TARGETS /// **lats, rhomboids, traps (primary); biceps, abs (secondary)**
EQUIPMENT /// **resistance band**

BANDED LAT PULL-DOWN

This exercise targets all of the muscles that contribute to a wide, beautiful back and a strong v-taper. The result is the appearance of a smaller waist and better balance between upper- and lower-body musculature. Banded lat pull-downs can also help improve pull-up strength and increase strength for big compound lifts like squats and deadlifts.

[1] Secure the resistance band over the top of a door or loop it over a tall, sturdy object. (Make sure both sides are even as this will ensure equal resistance on both sides.) Kneel as close as possible to the point where the band is anchored, and then grasp the ends of the band with a neutral grip. Pull down slightly to create tension in the band.

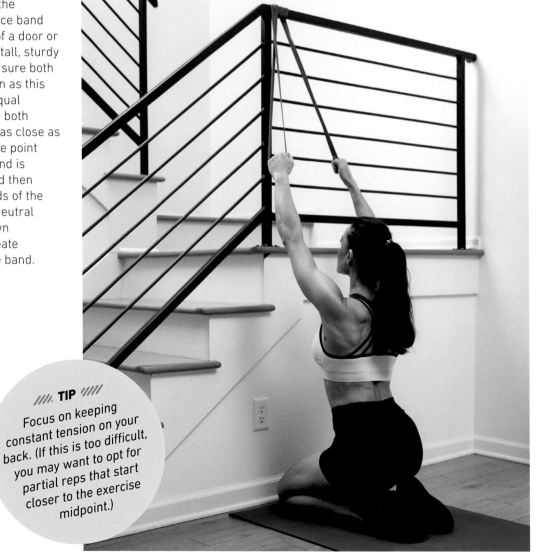

//// **TIP** ////
Focus on keeping constant tension on your back. (If this is too difficult, you may want to opt for partial reps that start closer to the exercise midpoint.)

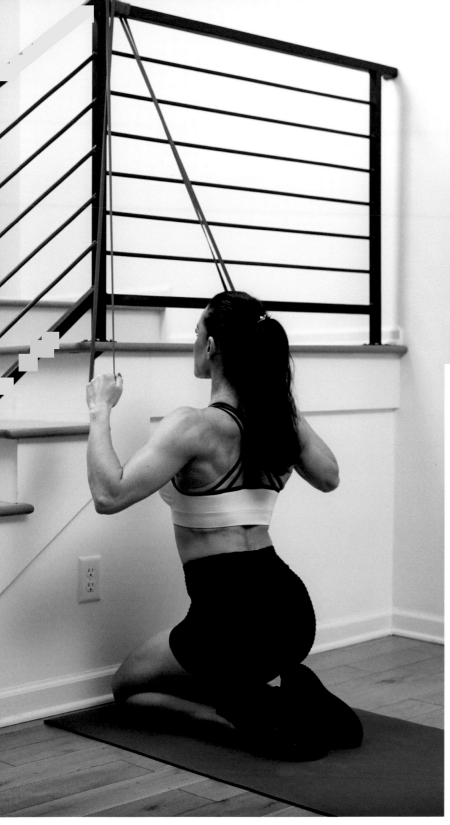

[2] Keeping your elbows in-line with your body, pull the ends of the band down toward your shoulder. Pause briefly before extending your arms back up to the starting point.

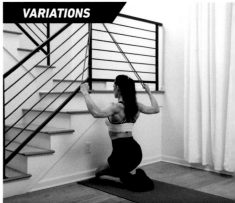

WIDE-GRIP PULL-DOWN Kneel under the point where the band is secured and grasp the ends with an overhand grip that's about twice shoulder width. Pull the ends downward so they're in a straight line with your upper body.

SINGLE-ARM PULL-DOWN Extend your nonworking arm upward and grasp the band at a high point, keeping the arm straight and the elbow locked. Grasp the other end of the band with the hand of your working arm, and then pull downward toward your shoulder. Repeat on the opposite side.

TARGETS /// **upper lats, rear delts, rhomboids (primary); traps, core (secondary)**
EQUIPMENT /// **resistance band**

BANDED HIGH ROW

Add this move to your routine if you're working on building a strong v-taper. Banded high rows add both detail and width across the upper back and rear delts. The result is the illusion of a smaller waist and also better balance between the upper and lower body. Rows also help improve posture as you stretch the chest during the movement and squeeze your shoulder blades together.

TRAIN THE RIGHT WAY

DO: Keep constant tension in the band.

DON'T: Rock with your upper body, which will engage the wrong muscles.

[**1**] Anchor a resistance band to a secure object at chest height. (Alternatively, you can place a resistance band around your feet while you're seated and your legs are extended.) Stand with soft knees and grasp the ends of the band with a neutral grip, ensuring that there is tension in the band when your arms are fully extended. (If you're standing, step away from the anchor point to add tension in the band. If you're seated, wrap the bands around your feet to add tension.)

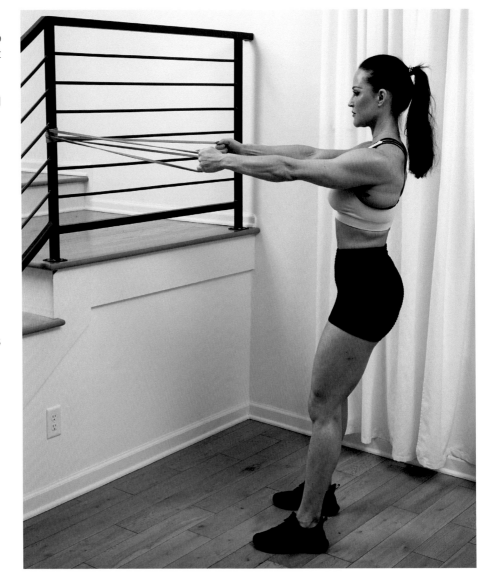

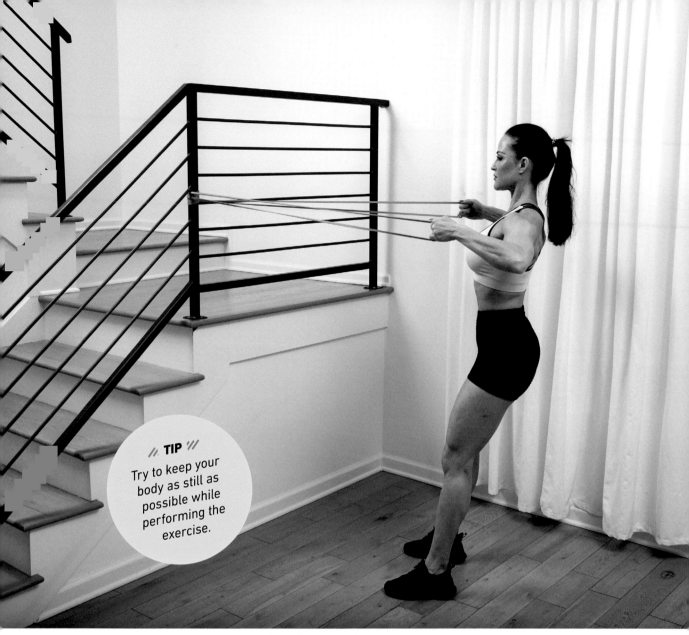

// TIP //

Try to keep your body as still as possible while performing the exercise.

[■] Lean back slightly, and pull the ends of the band to your chest, keeping your elbows pointed outward. Pause slightly at mid rep, and then control the tempo as you extend your arms back to the starting position.

VARIATIONS

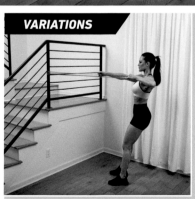

SINGLE-ARM HIGH ROW Grasp the ends of the band with an overhand grip. Keeping one arm stationary, perform all reps on one side. Repeat on the opposite side, making sure that you use the same form and perform equal reps on each side.

TARGETS /// **rhomboids, traps, lats (primary); biceps (secondary)**
EQUIPMENT /// **yoga mat, resistance band**

SEATED BANDED ROW

A strong back not only enhances strength in compound lifts, it creates width across the upper body. The key to effectively training the back is to slow down the tempo, keep tension on the muscles, and do a variety of rows and pull-downs. The banded row gives you the most "bang for the buck" of all row variations as it hits the greatest number of muscles in the back.

TRAIN THE RIGHT WAY

DO: Pull through the elbows and keep your forearms parallel to the floor.

DON'T: Lean back too much, as the emphasis can shift to the lower back.

[1] Sit on the floor with your legs fully extended and your back straight. Wrap the resistance band around the bottoms of your feet. Grasp the ends of the band using a neutral grip. Keeping your arms fully extended, lean back slightly to add tension in the band.

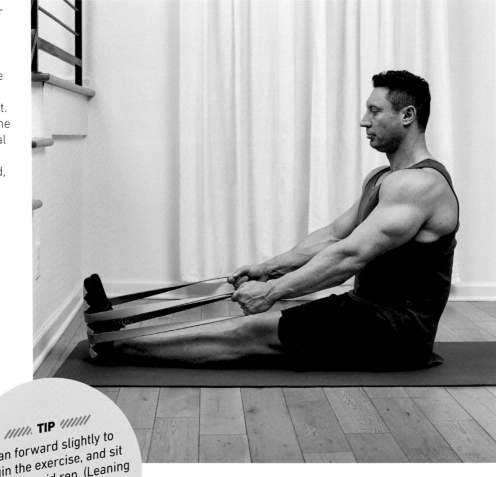

///// **TIP** /////
Lean forward slightly to begin the exercise, and sit upright at mid rep. (Leaning back too much will engage the lower back.)

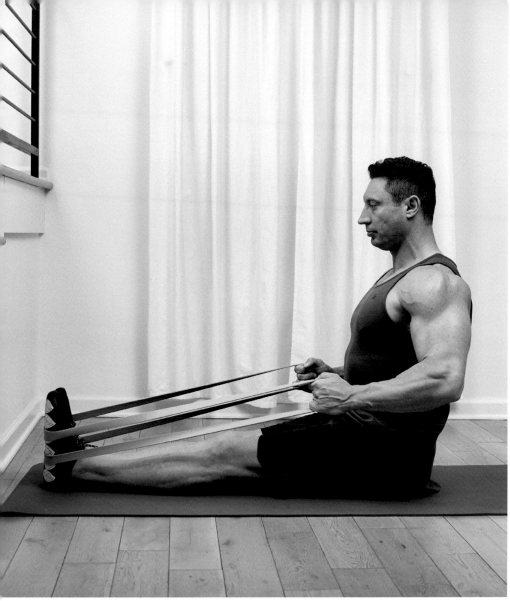

[2] Sit tall and engage your core. Extend your shoulders forward slightly, and pull the ends of the band in toward your stomach. (As you pull, rotate your shoulders back.) Pull through a comfortable, full range of motion and pause mid rep while squeezing your shoulder blades together. Using your back, slowly release the band back to the starting position.

VARIATIONS

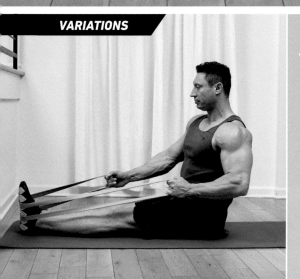

SINGLE-ARM BANDED ROW Grasp the ends of the band and perform all reps on your nondominant side first, leaving the nonworking arm straight and using it to secure the band. Repeat on the opposite side. (This variation is great for balancing the physique.)

WIDE-GRIP BANDED ROW Extend your arms and separate your hands to about one and a half times shoulder width. Keep your hands at this width and perform the exercise as instructed.

TARGETS /// **lats, chest, triceps (primary); abs (secondary)**
EQUIPMENT /// **bench, dumbbell**

DUMBBELL PULL-OVER

While many training programs feature compound movements, the pull-over is an isolation movement with too many benefits to ignore. It's one of the few exercises that simultaneously trains opposing muscle groups: the back and chest. It's also a movement that can improve spine health and bolster stability. Perform a full range of motion with this exercise, and you'll improve your upper body flexibility.

TRAIN THE RIGHT WAY

DO: Inhale as you lower the dumbbell, and focus on using just your lats.

DON'T: Allow your back to over arch.

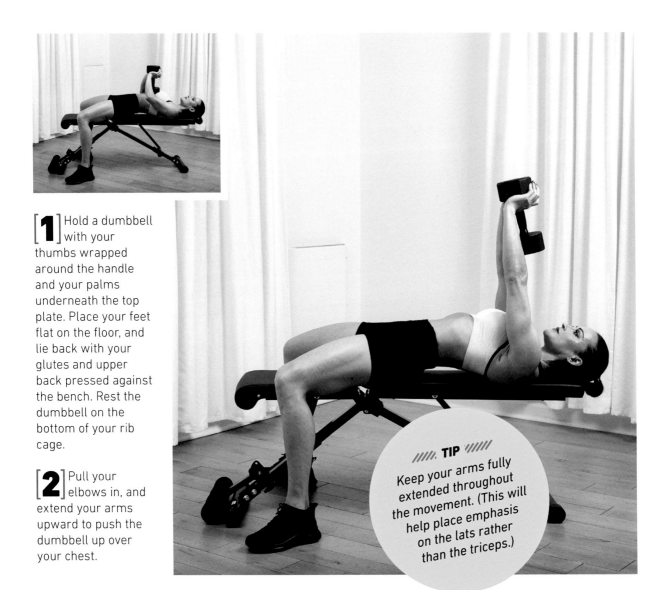

[1] Hold a dumbbell with your thumbs wrapped around the handle and your palms underneath the top plate. Place your feet flat on the floor, and lie back with your glutes and upper back pressed against the bench. Rest the dumbbell on the bottom of your rib cage.

[2] Pull your elbows in, and extend your arms upward to push the dumbbell up over your chest.

///// **TIP** /////
Keep your arms fully extended throughout the movement. (This will help place emphasis on the lats rather than the triceps.)

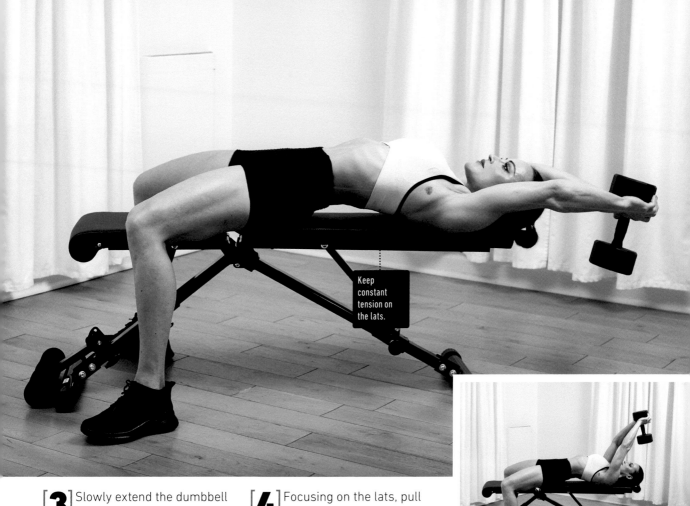

Keep constant tension on the lats.

[3] Slowly extend the dumbbell back and downward behind your head, pausing when you feel a stretch in your lats.

[4] Focusing on the lats, pull the dumbbell back up to a point just before your arms reach perpendicular to the floor.

VARIATIONS

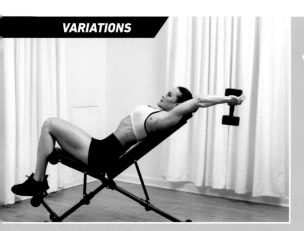

INCLINE DUMBBELL PULL-OVER (MORE CHALLENGING) Set your bench to a 45-degree angle, and perform the exercise as instructed.

SINGLE-ARM DUMBBELL PULL-OVER Hold a light dumbbell in one hand, and perform the exercise as instructed. Complete all reps on one side and then switch to the opposite side.

BANDED STRAIGHT-ARM PUSH-DOWN Secure a resistance band at the top of a door, and stand 2 to 3 feet from the door. Using an overhand grip on the band, straighten your arms starting at around shoulder height, and then push the bands down toward your knees.

TARGETS /// **lats, traps, rear delts (primary); biceps, glutes (secondary)**
EQUIPMENT /// **dumbbells**

YATES ROW

Build width in your upper back with this exercise created by legendary bodybuilder Dorian Yates. You'll perform this row with a more upright stance, which will hit all the muscles in the upper back. The result will be a beautifully tapered back that creates the illusion of a smaller waist. Since you'll be standing more upright than you would be with a traditional bent over row, you'll lessen the risk of lower back strain.

TRAIN THE RIGHT WAY

DO: Keep your elbows close to your sides and your forearms straight down.

DON'T: Use momentum to pull the dumbbells, which will train muscle groups other than the targeted muscle groups.

[**1**] Grasp the dumbbells with an underhand grip and position them in front of you at about shoulder width. Stand with your feet about shoulder width apart, bend forward at the hips, and keep your back flat.

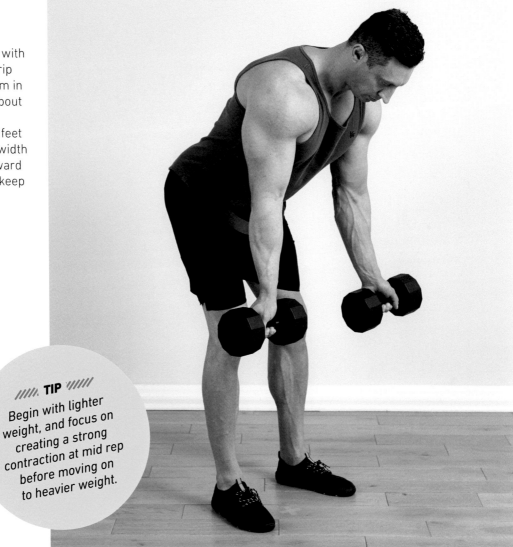

///// **TIP** /////
Begin with lighter weight, and focus on creating a strong contraction at mid rep before moving on to heavier weight.

[2] Pull the dumbbells up toward your hip bones, rotating your shoulders back and down and squeezing your shoulder blades together as you pull, and then control the weight back to the starting position.

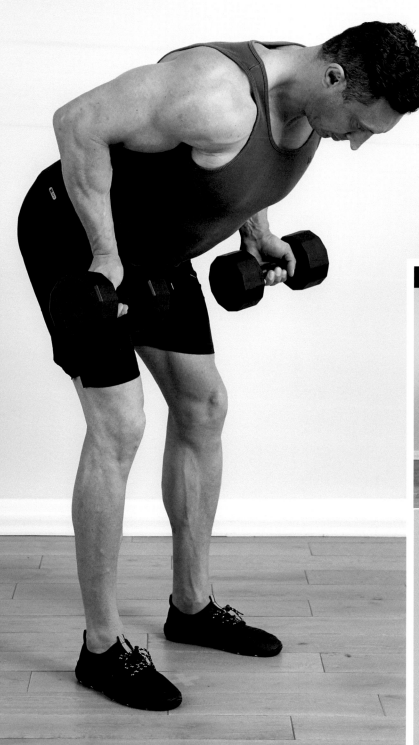

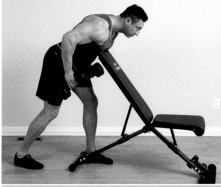

VARIATIONS

HELMS ROW Grasp dumbbells with a neutral grip, and face the high side of an incline bench. Place your chest on top of the bench with one leg forward and one leg back in a staggered position. Round your upper back over the bench slightly, and pull the dumbbells upward, keeping your elbows in as you pull.

BANDED LOW ROW Secure a resistance band toward the bottom of a door or other sturdy ground-level object. Using an underhand grip, back away to create tension in the band, and then pull the band toward your hip bones.

TARGETS /// lats, rhomboids, traps (primary); lower back, biceps (secondary)
EQUIPMENT /// bench, dumbbells

SUPINE DUMBBELL ROW

Building width and density in the upper-middle back can be challenging at home. This exercise does the job well, and using a bench adds additional core support and limits the use of momentum which can be a drawback. Unlike machines that can allow for an uneven pull between left and right sides, dumbbells ensure an even pull on both sides which, over time, contributes to muscle symmetry.

TRAIN THE RIGHT WAY

DO: Keep your wrists straight and squeeze your shoulder blades together at the top of the exercise.

DON'T: Shrug the weights first as this will recruit mostly the traps.

[1] Adjust the bench to a 45-degree angle. Lie stomach down on the bench, grasping the dumbbells with a neutral grip and allowing your arms to hang straight down. Plant both feet solidly on the floor to create a strong foundation. Pull your chest up slightly.

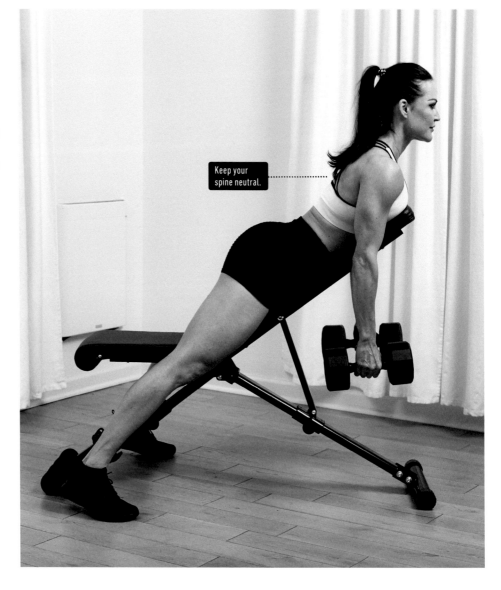

Keep your spine neutral.

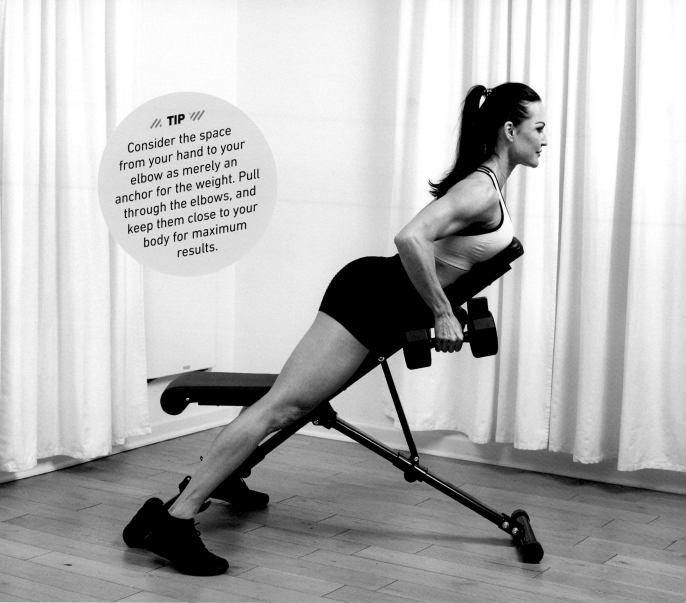

[2] Pull the dumbbells upward and slightly back, focusing on leading the exercise with your elbows. Pause slightly at the top of the rep, and then slowly lower the dumbbells back down to the starting point. (Don't pause at the bottom of the rep.)

VARIATIONS

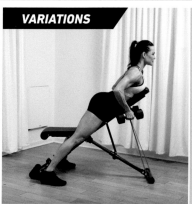

BANDED SUPINE ROW (MORE CHALLENGING) Secure a band to the bottom and toward the front of the bench and opposite the seat. Perform the exercise with resistance bands or add resistance bands to the dumbbell exercise for increased resistance.

HIGH-INCLINE SUPINE ROW Adjust the bench to a 60-degree angle. Perform the exercise as instructed. (This variation hits the upper lats, rhomboids, and rear delts.)

TARGETS /// **middle lats, rhomboids, traps (primary); biceps, forearms (secondary)**
EQUIPMENT /// **bench, dumbbell**

SINGLE-ARM DUMBBELL ROW

You can create width and definition in your middle back with rows. As one of the six basic lifts, rows should be a staple in any bodybuilding program. This single-arm exercise helps create muscle balance from the right side to the left side. It can improve overall pulling strength and help prevent injury. Rows tend to be easier on the shoulders than pull-downs, so adding this exercise and its variations will help build muscle in a more sustainable way.

TRAIN THE RIGHT WAY

DO: Keep constant tension on the back throughout the exercise, and don't rest at the bottom of the rep.

DON'T: Allow your shoulder on the working side to rise above parallel to the ground.

[**1**] Grasp a dumbbell with your nondominant hand and place your opposite hand and knee on the bench. Position your other leg underneath your body with your foot flat on the floor. Extend your working arm downward, holding the dumbbell with a neutral grip.

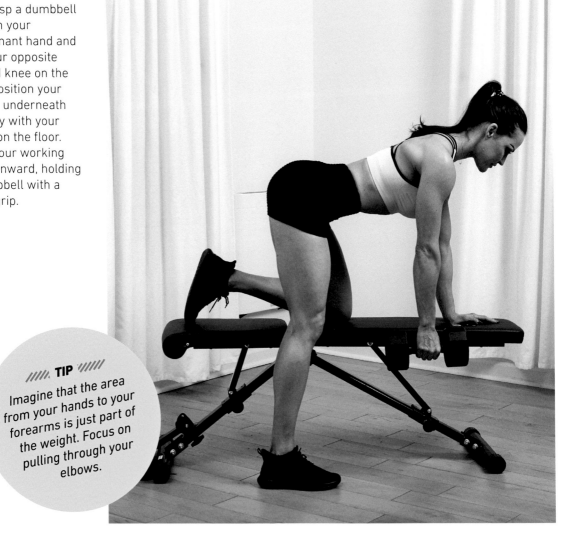

///// **TIP** /////
Imagine that the area from your hands to your forearms is just part of the weight. Focus on pulling through your elbows.

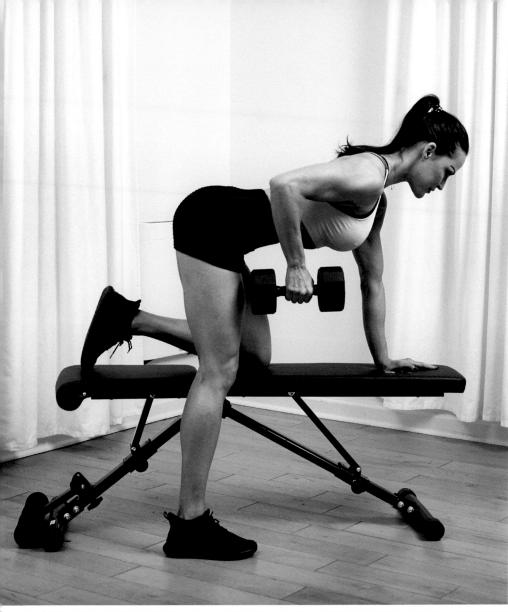

[2] With your shoulders parallel to the floor, your back flat, and your neck in a neutral position, pull the dumbbell up to your waistline, keeping your elbow close to your rib cage as you pull. Slowly lower the dumbbell back down to the starting position. Repeat on the opposite side.

VARIATIONS

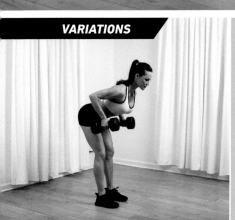

BENT OVER ROW Stand with your feet shoulder width apart, and hinge forward at the hips until your upper body is just above parallel to the floor. Hold a dumbbell in each hand, and allow your arms to extend downward while keeping your back flat and core tight. Using just your back, pull the dumbbells up to your waistline. (The grip can be underhand, neutral, or overhand.)

LOW-INCLINE DUMBBELL ROW Adjust the bench one peg higher than flat to create a low incline. Place your knee on the flat seat and then place your nonworking hand on the inclined portion of the bench. Perform the exercise as instructed. (This variation hits the area higher on the back.)

TARGETS /// **lats, traps, rear delts (primary); biceps (secondary)**
EQUIPMENT /// **resistance band**

BANDED LOW ROW

Strengthen your back and shoulders, improve scapular retraction, and improve shoulder health with this exercise. You can secure the resistance band in a doorframe or secure it to a sturdy anchor point. Since you're working with resistance bands, focus on keeping your tempo slow around the mid-rep point to help build width across your back and rear delts.

TRAIN THE RIGHT WAY

DO: Keep your wrists unbroken and pull through your elbows.

DON'T: Use momentum, which can cause other muscles to take over.

[1] Secure a resistance band in a door frame or to a sturdy object at about mid-shin height. Stand with your feet shoulder width apart with soft knees and an engaged core. Grasp the ends of the resistance band with a neutral grip that is positioned at just about the width of your shoulders. Lean back from the band enough to create tension, while still keeping your arms extended.

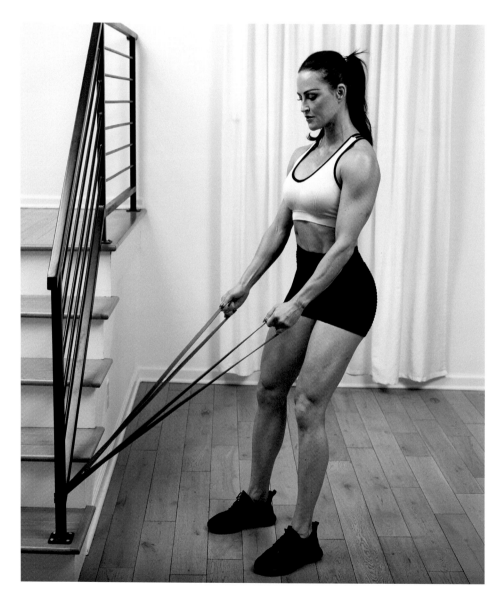

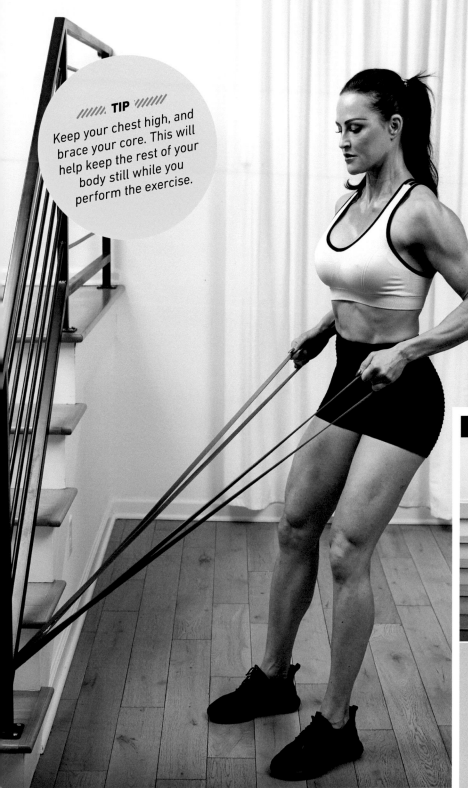

TIP

Keep your chest high, and brace your core. This will help keep the rest of your body still while you perform the exercise.

[2] Pull the band up toward your abdomen, rotating your shoulders back and down and squeezing your shoulder blades together as you pull. Pause briefly, and then slowly extend your arms back to the starting position.

VARIATIONS

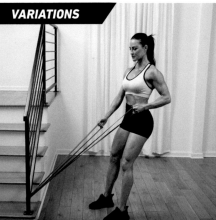

SINGLE-ARM LOW ROW Get into position as instructed. While one arm remains extended, perform all reps on one side and then repeat on the opposite side. (Use your nonworking arm to add tension in the band and to keep it from sliding.)

TARGETS **///** **lats, rhomboids, traps, core (primary);**
biceps, forearms (secondary)
EQUIPMENT **///** **dumbbells**

RENEGADE ROW

Build your back, strengthen your core, and improve coordination and balance with this dynamic exercise. While the main focus of renegade rows is the lats, it's considered a total body exercise since you'll be stabilizing yourself with almost every muscle in your body. Renegade rows can also be used as a metabolic movement—simply go lighter with the dumbbells and increase your reps.

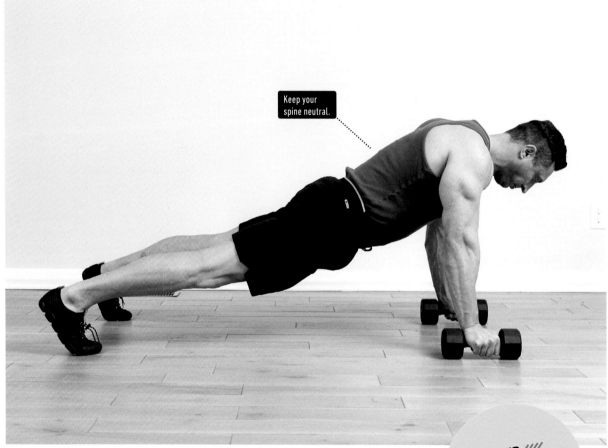

Keep your spine neutral.

[**1**] Place two dumbbells on the floor about shoulder width apart. Grasp the dumbbells and drop down into a high plank position with your feet positioned slightly wider than shoulder width apart.

/// TIP ///
Placing your feet a bit wider will help with stabilization.

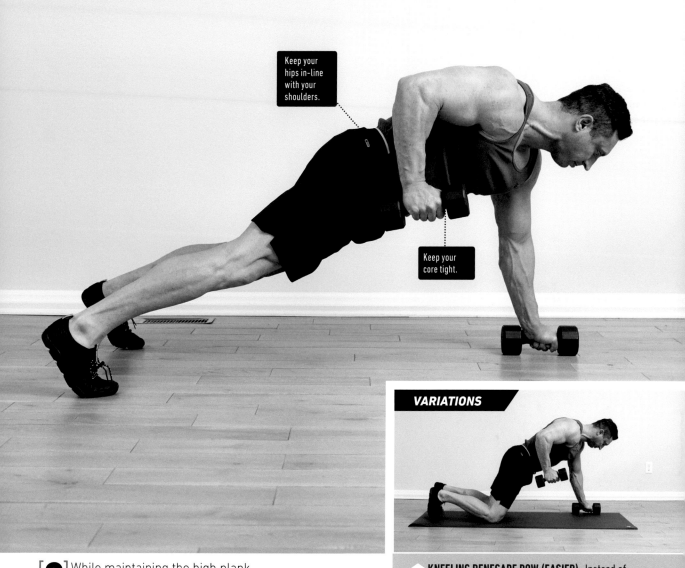

Keep your hips in-line with your shoulders.

Keep your core tight.

VARIATIONS

2 While maintaining the high plank position, slowly pull one dumbbell up toward your ribcage, and then slowly lower the dumbbell back down to the floor, making sure you remain balanced. Repeat the movement on the other side.

KNEELING RENEGADE ROW (EASIER) Instead of getting into plank position, place your knees on the floor, and then flatten your back. Perform the move while balanced on your knees. (This variation is easier and can be a good starting variation for beginners.)

RENEGADE ROW TO PUSH-UP (MORE CHALLENGING) Perform the renegade row as instructed, but after performing a row on each side, lower your body to the floor and then push back up. This variation hits the chest and is a great cardio move.

TARGETS /// **lats, rhomboids, traps (primary); biceps, core (secondary)**
EQUIPMENT /// **resistance band**

SINGLE-ARM SIDE PULL-DOWN

If you ever played sports or worked in a trade, chances are one side of your body is more developed than the other. Unilateral, or single-arm, exercises like this one can help even out asymmetries that can naturally develop from being either left- or right-handed. Not only will this improve aesthetics but it also can prevent injury. This exercise is simple to set up, but it's far from easy to execute!

TRAIN THE RIGHT WAY

DO: Mirror the motion and stance on each side to ensure you get even results on both sides.

DON'T: Allow the band to become slack at any point during the exercise as you will stop working the muscles.

[**1**] Grasp a resistance band with your nonworking arm, leaving a short segment of the band just above one end. Extend your nonworking arm directly overhead, locking out your arm, and then grasp the loop at the short end with your working hand. Position your working arm in-line with your ear.

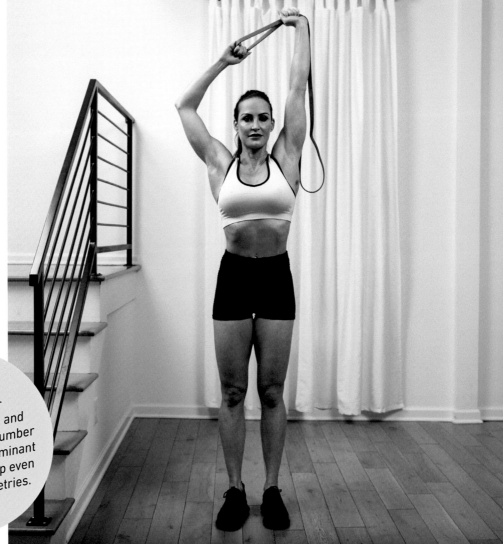

///// **TIP** /////
Begin with your nondominant arm, and then do the same number of reps on your dominant side. This will help even out any asymmetries.

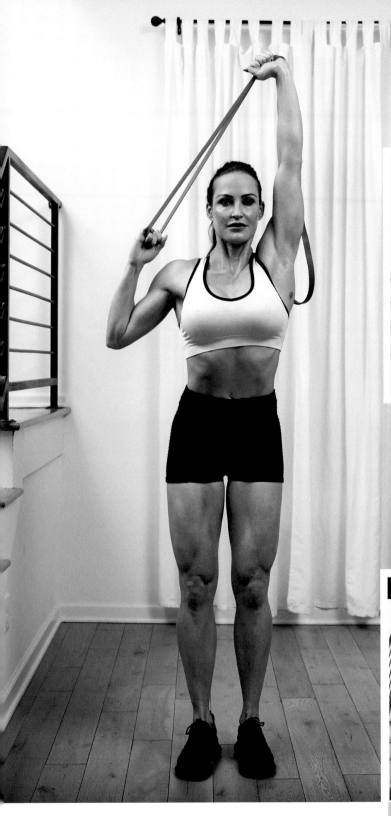

[2] Pull your working arm downward and outward until the upper arm is past parallel to the floor, squeezing your lat as you pull.

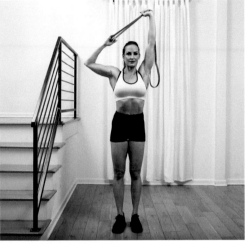

[3] Slowly control your arm back to just before the starting position, ensuring tension remains in the band. Perform the prescribed number of reps on one side, and then switch to the opposite side. (Make sure the resistance band segment is an equal length for both sides.)

VARIATIONS

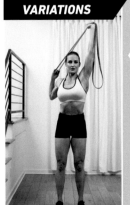

SINGLE-ARM PULL-DOWN
Extend your nonworking arm upward and then slightly out in front of you. Grasp the end of the band, and pull it down and slightly backward. (This variation targets more of the rear delts.)

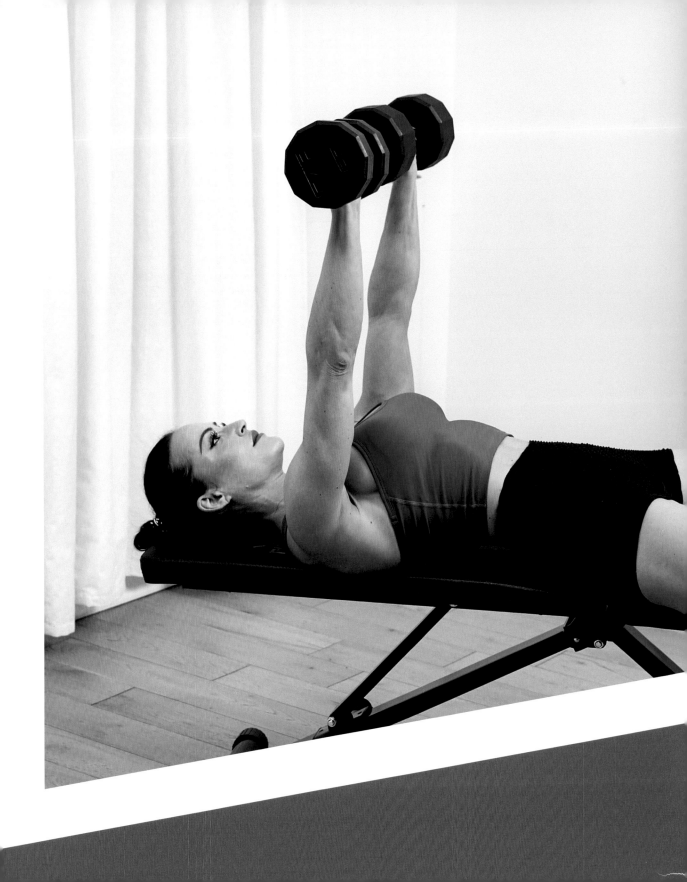

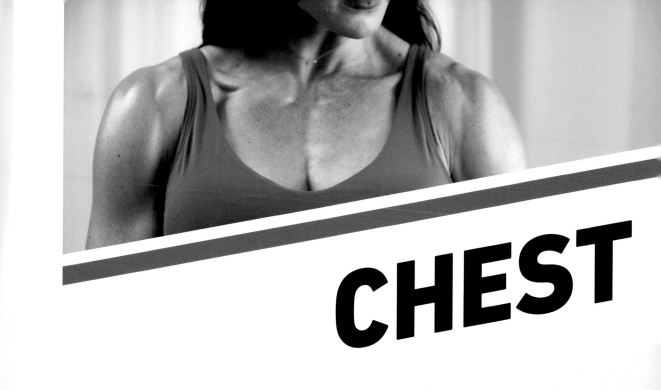

CHEST

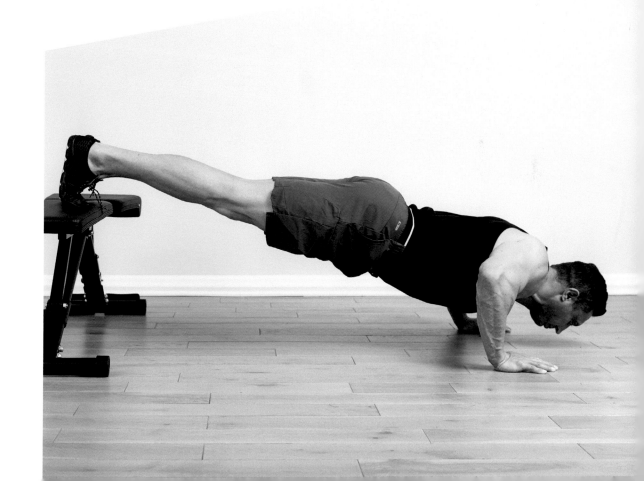

TARGETS /// **pectorals, front delts, triceps (primary); lats, abs (secondary)**
EQUIPMENT /// **bench, dumbbells**

DUMBBELL BENCH PRESS

The bench press is one of the six basic lifts. By incorporating it into your routine, you'll train not only your chest but also your shoulders, triceps, lats, and core. Mastering this lift will not only improve your upper body strength and power, but allow you to create many variations to further your progress as well. Using dumbbells will improve symmetry and is a much safer alternative to the barbell bench press.

[1] Sit on the end of the bench. Grasp the dumbbells and place them on the tops of each leg and just above the knees.

[2] Lie back on the bench, using your legs to "kick" each dumbbell up to the front of your shoulders as you recline. Once you're lying flat on the bench, press your glutes into the bench, place your feet flat on the floor, and pin your shoulder blades back and down.

[3] Push your elbows out to slowly maneuver the dumbbells outward until your upper arms are parallel to the floor and the dumbbells are just wider than shoulder width apart.

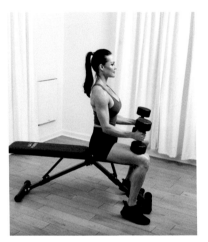
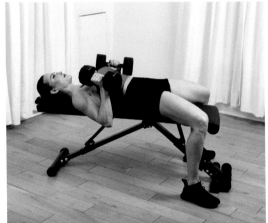
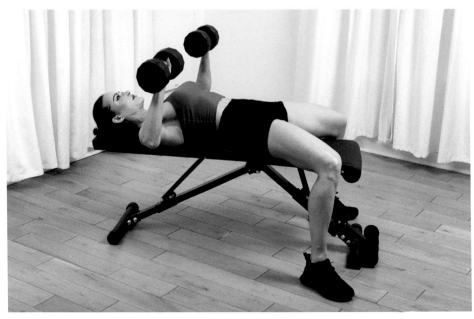

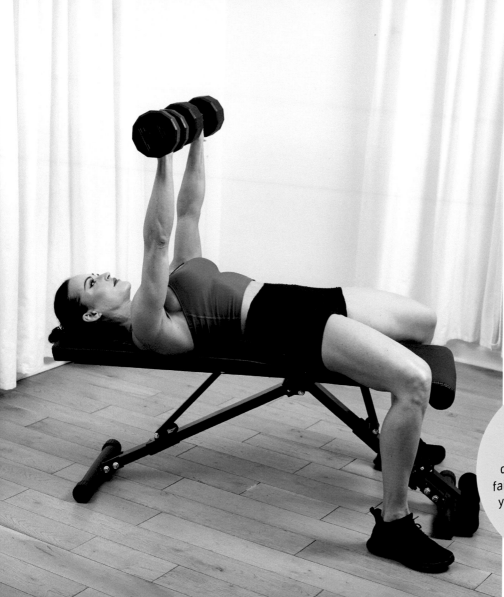

[**4**] Keeping your core tight, wrists straight, and elbows underneath the dumbbells, press the dumbbells upward and inward to bring them together at the top, and then bring them back down to the starting position at the bottom of the rep. (As you press, think about making a triangle with the range of motion.)

///// **TIP** /////
You can drop the dumbbells if you reach failure. You can also adjust your grip to a neutral grip if you experience wrist discomfort.

VARIATIONS

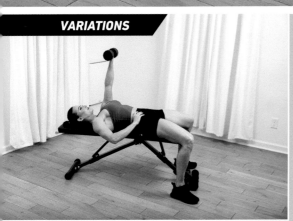

SINGLE-ARM DUMBBELL BENCH PRESS Choose a dumbbell that is 20 percent lighter than you'd normally use. Start with your nondominant side. Place your feet wider than normal, and counterbalance the movement with your opposite arm. Complete a set on one side, and then move to the other side.

BANDED BENCH PRESS (MORE CHALLENGING) Secure a resistance band with handles underneath the bench, ensuring that it's even on both sides. Lie back on the bench and grasp each end of the band. Perform the exercise as instructed. Focus on the mid-rep portion of the exercise, as this will give you the most tension. (You can also use dumbbells along with the band for increased difficulty.)

TARGETS /// **upper chest, front delts (primary); triceps, core (secondary)**
EQUIPMENT /// **bench, dumbbells**

DUMBBELL INCLINE BENCH PRESS

Lifters often focus on building round delts but frequently ignore the upper chest. A well-developed upper chest ties the shoulders to the rest of the physique and gives it a beautiful flow. Female lifters especially should work the upper chest as upper body fullness can be lost when you're leaning down. Both females and males can benefit from added musculature in the upper chest as it can balance the upper body with the lower body and make the waist look smaller.

TRAIN THE RIGHT WAY

DO: Make sure your elbows remain underneath the dumbbells.

DON'T: Arch your back as this can shift the movement to more of a flat bench exercise.

[**1**] Adjust the bench to a 45-degree angle, and sit on the end of the bench. Grasp the dumbbells, and place them on the tops of your legs and just above your knees.

[**2**] Using your legs, "kick" the dumbbells up to your shoulders as you lie back on the bench.

[**3**] Push your elbows out to slowly maneuver the dumbbells outward until your upper arms are parallel to the floor and the dumbbells are just wider than shoulder width apart.

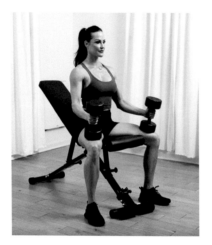

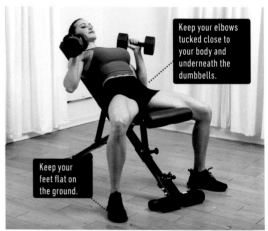

Keep your elbows tucked close to your body and underneath the dumbbells.

Keep your feet flat on the ground.

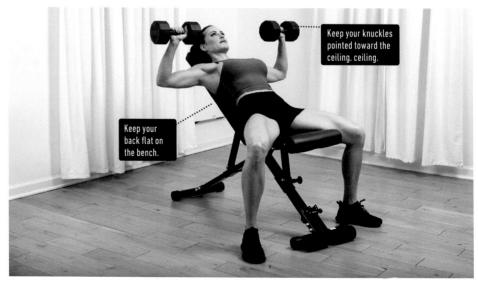

Keep your knuckles pointed toward the ceiling. ceiling.

Keep your back flat on the bench.

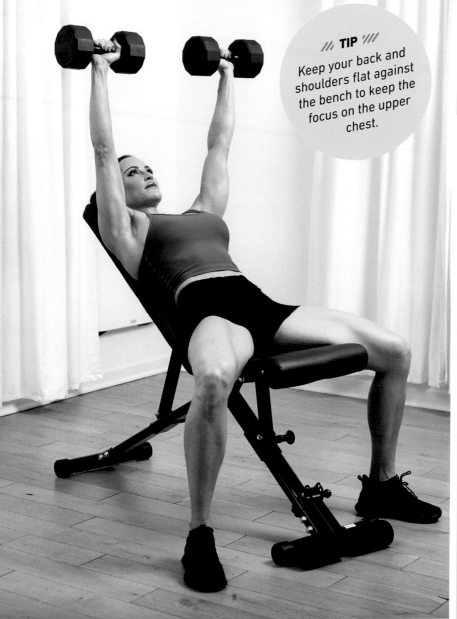

/// TIP ///

Keep your back and shoulders flat against the bench to keep the focus on the upper chest.

VARIATIONS

BANDED INCLINE BENCH PRESS (MORE CHALLENGING) Secure a resistance band underneath the bench with equal length on each side. Grasp the band as you lean back on the bench, and place your feet firmly on the floor. Press the band upward just as you would with dumbbells. Focus your efforts on the midrange portion of the rep as this is where you'll get the most tension.

HIGH INCLINE BENCH PRESS Adjust the bench to 60 to 75 degrees. (The higher the incline, the higher on the chest you will work.) Use a lighter weight than you'd use for traditional incline bench, and perform the exercise as instructed. (This variation is effective for building muscle just under the collarbone and for building the front delts.)

SINGLE-DUMBBELL INCLINE BENCH PRESS Place each hand around each end of one dumbbell, and hold it so it's parallel to the floor. Perform the exercise as instructed. (This will give you a narrow grip and will work more of your upper-mid chest and triceps.)

[4] Keeping your core tight, wrists straight, and elbows underneath the dumbbells, press the dumbbells upward and inward to bring them together at the top, and then bring them back down to the starting position. (As you press, think about making a triangle shape with the range of motion.)

TARGETS /// **pectorals, front delts, triceps (primary); lats, abs (secondary)**
EQUIPMENT /// **bench, dumbbells**

DUMBBELL INCLINE SQUEEZE PRESS

This unconventional bench press variation effectively targets and isolates the chest and may quickly become your favorite lift for the chest. The dumbbells remain in contact with each other as you press and lower them through the range of motion, resulting in constant tension and an incredible pump. And since this exercise uses lighter weights than would be used for a traditional bench press, it may be a good substitute for those with shoulder issues.

TRAIN THE RIGHT WAY

DO: Keep your wrists straight and actively press the dumbbells together throughout the exercise.

DON'T: Use a false grip for this exercise. Your thumbs are necessary to help stabilize the dumbbells.

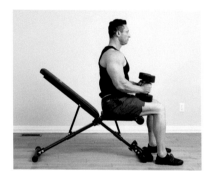

[1] Adjust the bench to a 45- to 60-degree angle. Sit on the end of the bench. Grasp the dumbbells with a neutral grip, and set them on their ends on top of your quads. (Go with lighter weight than you would if you were using a flat bench for the squeeze press.)

[2] As you lie back, use your legs to "kick" the dumbbells up to rest on your middle chest. Flare your elbows out and actively press the dumbbells together. (The dumbbells should be touching before you begin the exercise.)

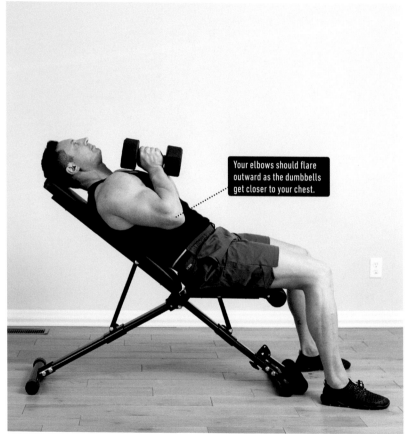

Your elbows should flare outward as the dumbbells get closer to your chest.

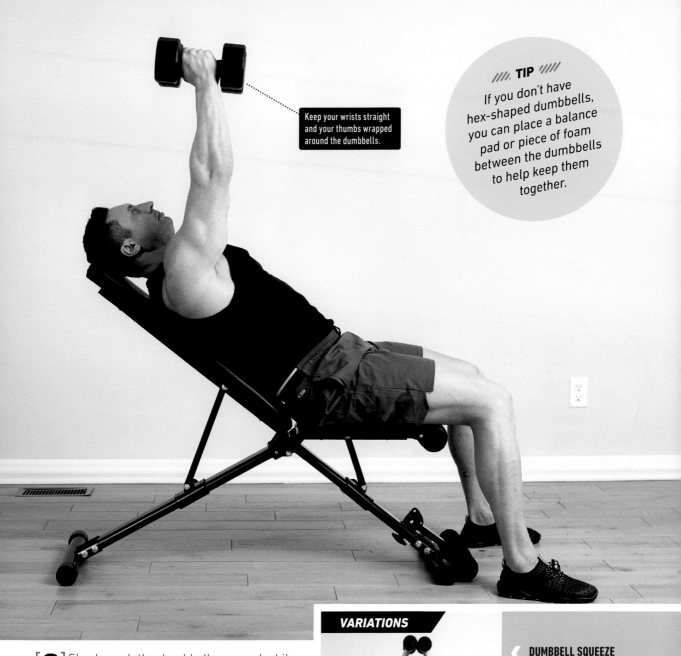

Keep your wrists straight and your thumbs wrapped around the dumbbells.

//// **TIP** ////

If you don't have hex-shaped dumbbells, you can place a balance pad or piece of foam between the dumbbells to help keep them together.

[3] Slowly push the dumbbells upward while simultaneously pressing them together as you push. Keep your core tight as you press, and slowly exhale as you push. Pause slightly when your arms are fully extended, and then slowly lower the dumbbells back down to a point just above your chest.

VARIATIONS

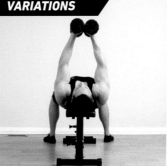

DUMBBELL SQUEEZE PRESS Use a flat bench, and go heavier than you would for the dumbbell incline squeeze press. Perform the exercise as instructed. (This variation hits the mid chest.)

TARGETS /// **upper chest, front delts (primary); triceps, core (secondary)**
EQUIPMENT /// **bench**

DECLINE PUSH-UP

Bodyweight exercises are the ultimate test of strength and technique, and they tend to hit multiple muscle groups that also carry over into everyday activities. One of the more difficult exercises, the decline push-up, hits all the upper body muscles required for generating pressing strength, and it also trains the core. You can adjust the angle of this exercise to make it easier or more difficult.

TRAIN THE RIGHT WAY

DO: Keep your elbows close to your body rather than allowing them to flare out.

DON'T: Allow your hips to sag, as this can cause stress on your lower back.

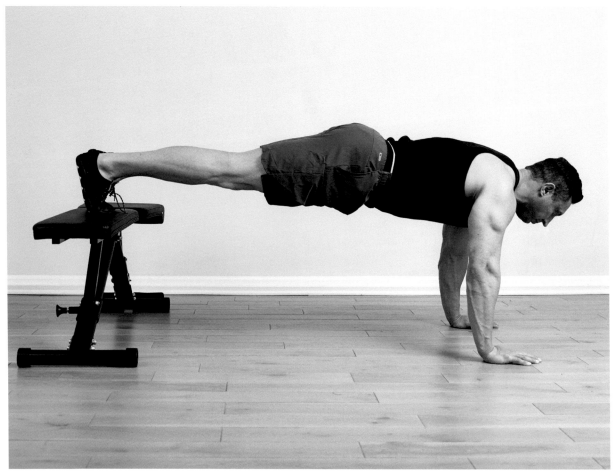

[**1**] Place your toes on the bench, and then drop down into a plank position with your arms positioned shoulder width apart and your hands flat on the floor.

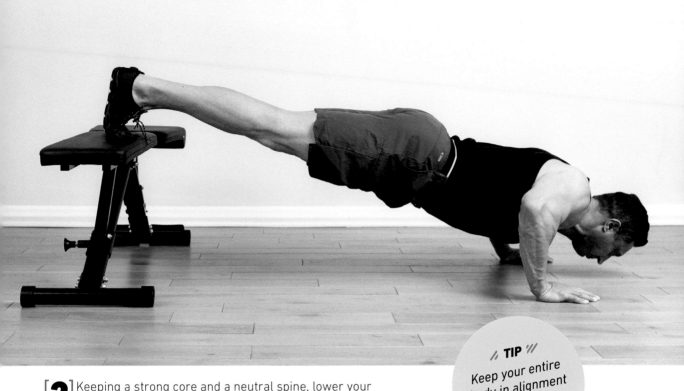

[2] Keeping a strong core and a neutral spine, lower your upper body down to the floor, and then use your chest, shoulders, and triceps to press yourself back up to the starting position.

// TIP //

Keep your entire body in alignment throughout the exercise.

VARIATIONS

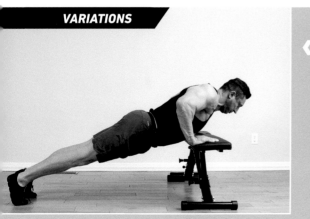

INCLINE PUSH-UP (EASIER) Get into a plank position with your hands on the bench and your toes on the floor. (Your hands should be positioned about shoulder width apart.) Slowly lower your body down toward the bench, pause just before your chest touches the bench, and then press yourself back up to the starting position.

DECLINE CLOSE-GRIP PUSH-UP (MORE CHALLENGING) Place your toes on the bench and your hands positioned close together on the floor. Perform the exercise as instructed. (This variation is much more difficult than the others and targets the triceps.)

TARGETS /// **upper chest (primary); front delts, triceps, forearms (secondary)**
EQUIPMENT /// **bench, dumbbells**

DUMBBELL INCLINE FLYE

While compound movements allow you to add muscle to multiple areas simultaneously, isolation exercises allow you to carefully sculpt your physique. They're also great for improving your mind-muscle connection. Dumbbell incline flyes target the upper chest specifically. Pairing them with the incline bench press will enable you to add some fullness to an area that tends to look flat when the delts are developed.

DO: Keep constant tension on the muscles by stopping just before your arms reach perpendicular to the floor.

DON'T: Overbend your elbows. This can shorten the lever of the exercise and allow other muscles to take over.

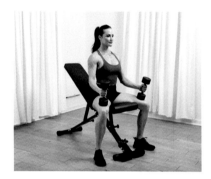

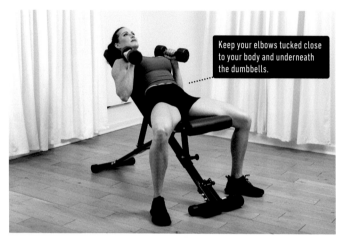

Keep your elbows tucked close to your body and underneath the dumbbells.

[**1**] Adjust the bench to a 45-degree angle. Sit fully on the bench with your feet placed flat on the floor. Rest the dumbbells on top of your quads using a neutral grip.

[**2**] Lie back on the bench, and use your legs to simultaneously "kick" the dumbbells up to a point between your front delts and collarbone.

[**3**] Come into the starting position by extending the dumbbells to a position just over your chin.

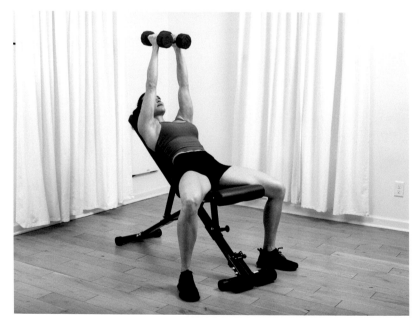

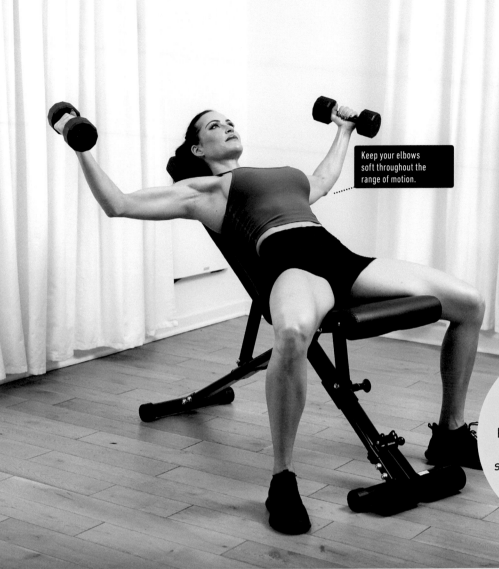

[4] Slowly lower the dumbbells out to your sides, pause when you feel a good stretch, and then press the dumbbells back up to the starting position.

Keep your elbows soft throughout the range of motion.

////// **TIP** //////
Picture yourself hugging a barrel. Your elbows should remain slightly bent throughout the exercise.

VARIATIONS

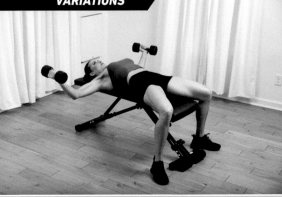

FLAT BENCH FLYE Set your bench to the flat position. Perform the exercise as instructed. (This variation will hit the middle chest.)

HIGH INCLINE FLYE Adjust your bench to a 60-degree angle, and perform the exercise as instructed. (This variation will hit higher up on the chest.)

TARGETS /// **chest, anterior delts (primary); triceps (secondary)**
EQUIPMENT /// **resistance band**

BANDED CROSS-BODY CHEST PRESS

The banded cross-body chest press allows you to target one side of the chest at a time and can help create strong curves that not only tie the shoulders in with the rest of your upper body but also give the appearance of a smaller waist.

TRAIN THE RIGHT WAY

DO: Keep your body straight on both sides when performing the exercise.

DON'T: Allow your hand to drift away from your body, which can cause other muscles to take over.

[1] Attach the resistance band to a door frame or other sturdy object at about shoulder height. Stand with your working side facing the band, and then grasp the end of the band using a neutral grip. Bend at the elbow to pull the band in front of your underarm. Step far enough away from the anchor point to create tension in the band and also allow a full range of motion.

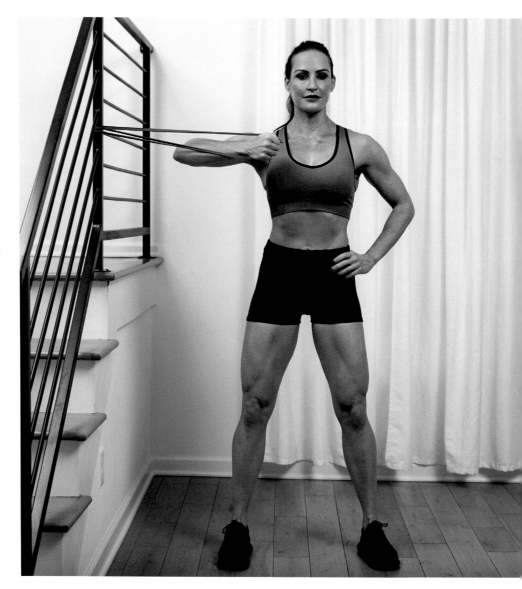

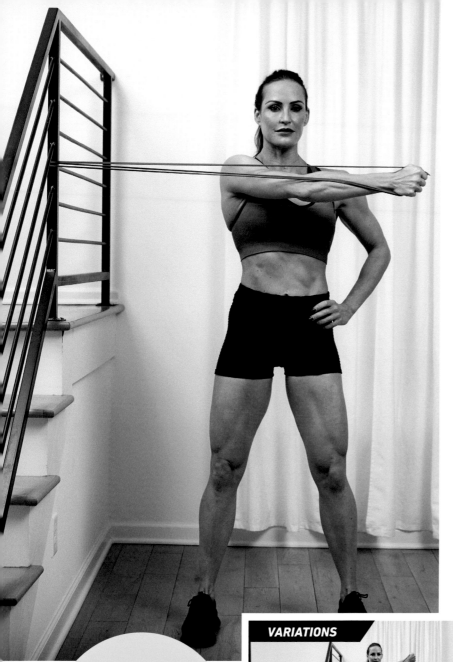

[2] Slowly press the band across the front of your body, keeping the range of motion parallel to the floor. Extend your arm fully while squeezing your chest.

[3] Slowly control the band back to a point just before the starting position to ensure you keep tension in the band. Perform the reps on one side, and then repeat the exercise on the opposite side, ensuring your form is a mirror image of the starting side.

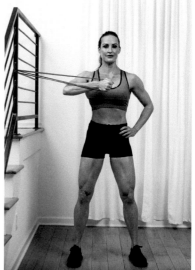

///// **TIP** /////
As you press, either watch or feel your muscle contract. This will strengthen your mind-muscle connection.

VARIATIONS

INCLINE CROSS-BODY CHEST PRESS Attach the band to a door frame or sturdy object at about knee height. Start with a bend in your elbow and a neutral grip. Press the band upward and across your body. Repeat on the opposite side. (This variation targets more of the upper chest and front delts.)

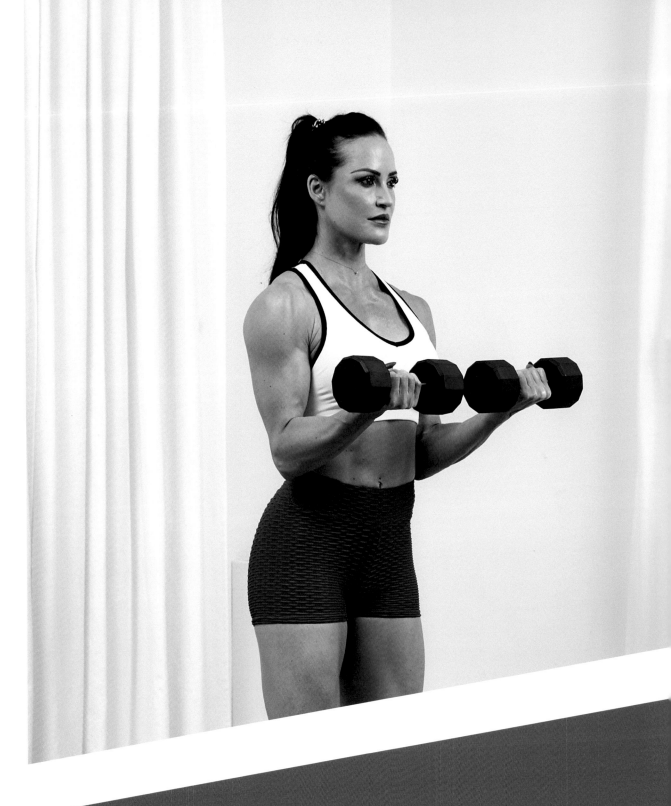

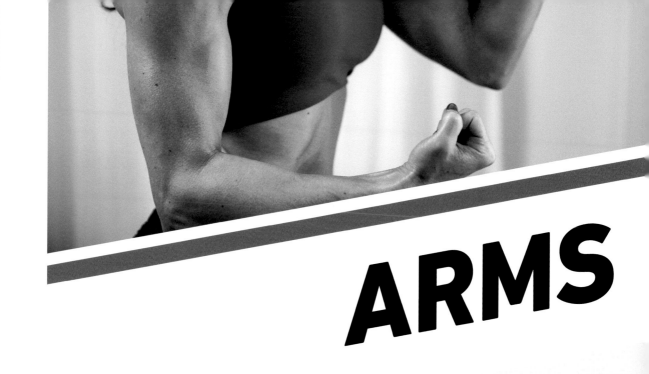

ARMS

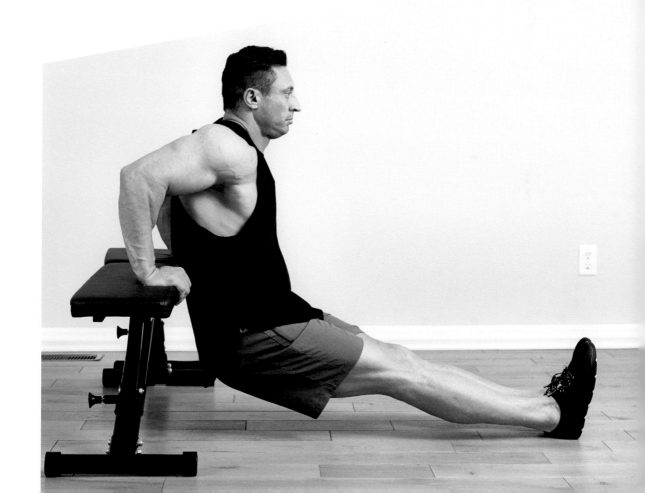

TARGETS /// **triceps (primary); lats, forearms (secondary)**
EQUIPMENT /// **dumbbells**

TRICEPS KICKBACK

You can build size and strength in your triceps by incorporating kickbacks into your training program. This movement focuses on the long head of the triceps, which can tie the arms together beautifully with the back of the shoulders. This is one of the most common exercises that are performed incorrectly, so stay focused during each rep to get maximum results.

TRAIN THE RIGHT WAY

DO: Keep your upper body still throughout the range of motion.

DON'T: Spend too time with your forearms perpendicular to the floor as you can lose tension on the triceps.

[1] Grasp two light dumbbells with a neutral grip. Lean forward at the hips until the upper body reaches almost parallel to the floor.

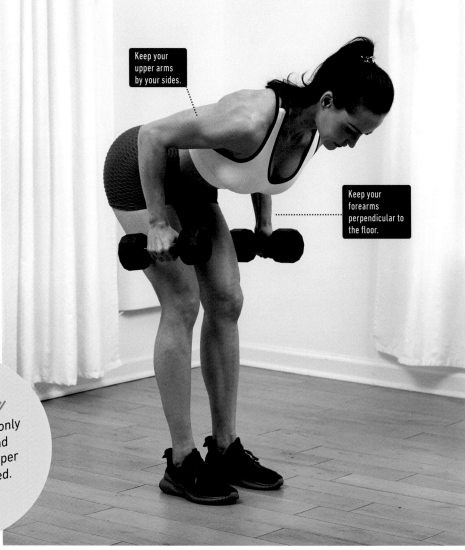

Keep your upper arms by your sides.

Keep your forearms perpendicular to the floor.

///// **TIP** /////
Focus on bending only at the elbow and keeping your upper arms stabilized.

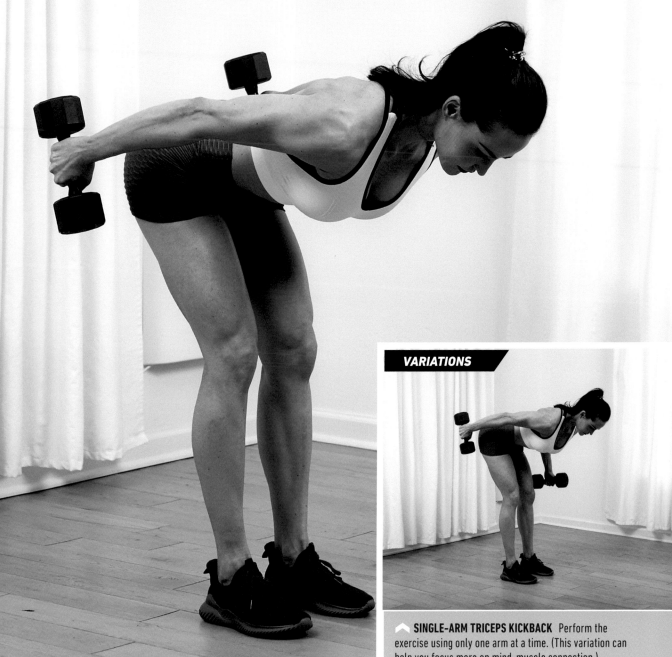

[2] Slowly push the dumbbells backward and upward until your arms are fully extended. At full extension, rotate your wrists inward slightly to accentuate the triceps more.

VARIATIONS

SINGLE-ARM TRICEPS KICKBACK Perform the exercise using only one arm at a time. (This variation can help you focus more on mind-muscle connection.)

INCLINE BENCH TRICEPS KICKBACK Adjust the bench to a 60-degree angle. Lie stomach down on the bench with your feet firmly planted on the floor. Grasp light dumbbells with a neutral grip, and lock your upper arms against your sides. Perform the exercise as instructed.

TARGETS /// **triceps (primary); chest, shoulders (secondary)**
EQUIPMENT /// **bench**

BENCH DIP

Many triceps-focused exercises are isolation movements, and while these can be great for adding detail, they don't do much for creating overall strength or for helping the physique flow together aesthetically. Bench dips are one of the few compound movements that will add strength and size to the triceps while also allowing the surrounding muscles to work in unison.

TRAIN THE RIGHT WAY

DO: Keep your body close to the bench.

DON'T: Allow your shoulders to shrug.

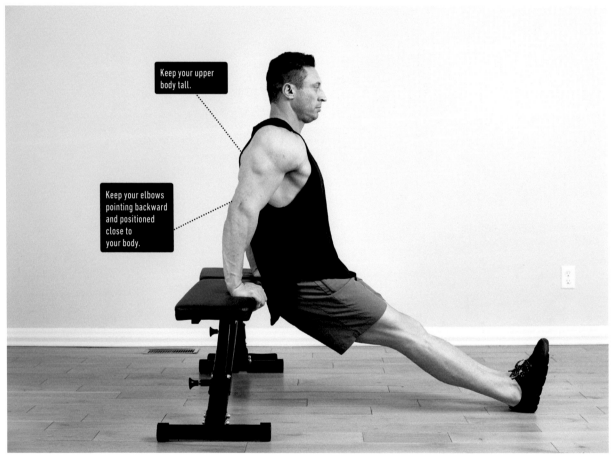

Keep your upper body tall.

Keep your elbows pointing backward and positioned close to your body.

[1] Sit on the side of the bench. Place your hands by your sides with your palms on the edge of the bench and your fingers facing forward. Extend your legs out in front of you with your weight centered in your heels. Keeping your arms extended, move your body about 1 inch (2.5cm) away from the edge of the bench.

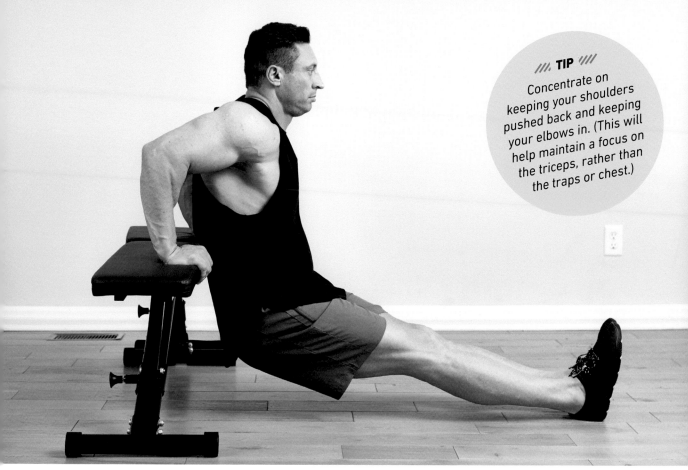

//// **TIP** ////

Concentrate on keeping your shoulders pushed back and keeping your elbows in. (This will help maintain a focus on the triceps, rather than the traps or chest.)

[2] Bend at the elbows to lower yourself down until you feel a stretch in your shoulders and chest. Pause and then use just your triceps to push yourself back up to the starting position.

VARIATIONS

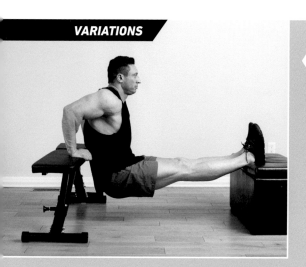

FEET-ELEVATED BENCH DIP (MORE CHALLENGING) This variation is great if you have a step stool or an extra chair at home. Place your bench close to the chair or step, and space them about one leg's length distance apart. Sit on the edge of the bench, and then place your heels on the step or chair with your legs fully extended. Perform the exercise as instructed.

WEIGHTED BENCH DIP (MORE CHALLENGING) Sit on the bench, and place a dumbbell on your lap and close to your hip crease. Place your feet on the floor with your legs just beyond perpendicular to the floor. Carefully prop yourself up onto your hands, and then move your body away from the bench far enough to clear it when you descend. (The range of motion is the same as standard bench dips, but be sure to keep your upper legs parallel to the floor to balance the weight.)

TARGETS /// **biceps (primary); front delts, forearms (secondary)**
EQUIPMENT /// **dumbbells**

STANDING BICEPS CURL

In the pursuit of building a complete physique, the arms can't be forgotten. Strong biceps can improve overall strength, especially when it comes to pulling exercises. The standing biceps curl is one of the most basic isolation movements, but with proper mind-muscle connection and technique, it can be a staple exercise for creating impressive biceps peaks.

TRAIN THE RIGHT WAY

DO: Keep tension on the muscle by not resting at the starting point and also stopping before your forearms are perpendicular to the floor.

DON'T: Use momentum to swing the weights through the range of motion as this can target other muscles.

[**1**] Stand with your feet shoulder width apart and with soft knees. Hold the dumbbells slightly in front of you using an underhand grip.

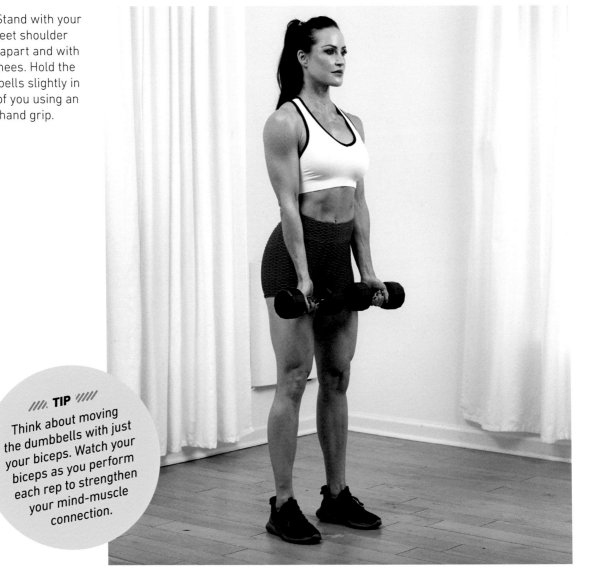

///. **TIP** ///
Think about moving the dumbbells with just your biceps. Watch your biceps as you perform each rep to strengthen your mind-muscle connection.

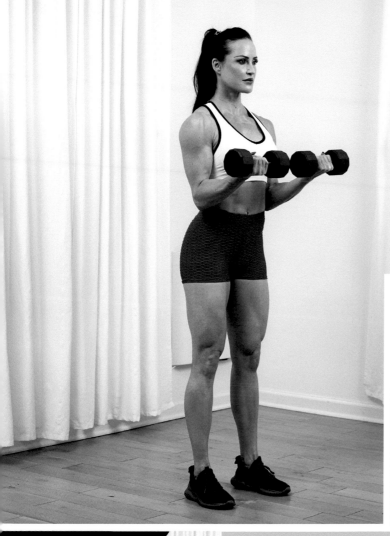

[2] With your upper arms pinned to your sides, your shoulders back, and your wrists straight, hinge at the elbows to pull the dumbbells upward and toward your chest by contracting the biceps. Pause just before your forearms reach perpendicular to the floor.

[3] Slowly lower the dumbbells back down to a point just before the starting position to maintain tension in the arms.

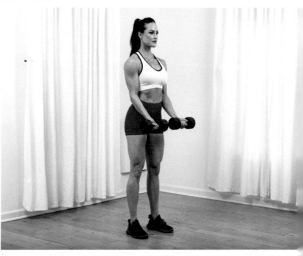

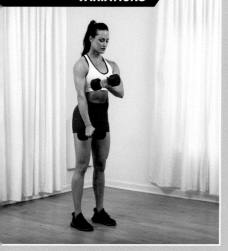

CROSS-BODY CURL Hold the dumbbells slightly out in front you with an overhand grip. One at a time and keeping your upper arms still, curl the dumbbells in an arc in front of your body while maintaining an overhand grip.

SEATED BICEPS CURL Sit on a flat bench with your feet together. Keep your upper arm stationary, and use an underhand grip. Hold your arms slightly away from your body to allow for a full range of motion.

SPIDER CURL Lie stomach-down on an incline bench set to 45 degrees. Hold the dumbbells with an underhand grip, and keep your upper arms perpendicular to the floor.

DUMBBELL PARTIAL-REP CURL Sit on a flat bench with your feet flat on the floor and slightly out in front of you. Hold the dumbbells just above your knees and with an underhand grip. Curl the dumbbells, stopping just before your forearms reach perpendicular at the top and just before the dumbbells touch your knees at the bottom. (This is great as a finisher or for a pump.)

DRAG CURL (MORE CHALLENGING) While standing, hold the dumbbells with an underhand grip and directly in front of your thighs. Drag the dumbbells upward. (A slight backward bend in the wrists will help you isolate the biceps.)

TARGETS /// **biceps (primary); front delts, forearms (secondary)**
EQUIPMENT /// **dumbbells**

BANDED BICEPS CURL

Add intensity to your biceps routine with banded biceps curls. Bands can create constant tension and be an effective substitute for cable exercises. When performing this exercise, it's key to focus on the mid-rep area of your range of motion as this is where the exercise will be the most difficult. This will also help give you the fastest results.

TRAIN THE RIGHT WAY

DO: Focus on maintaining tension on the biceps. If this means that your range of motion needs to be shortened compared to the dumbbell version, that's ok!

DON'T: Allow the band to go slack during the set.

[1] Stand with your feet shoulder width apart and with soft knees. Stand in the middle of the resistance band and grasp the band with an underhand grip and with your arms extended slightly out in front of you. Widen your stance to create tension in the band.

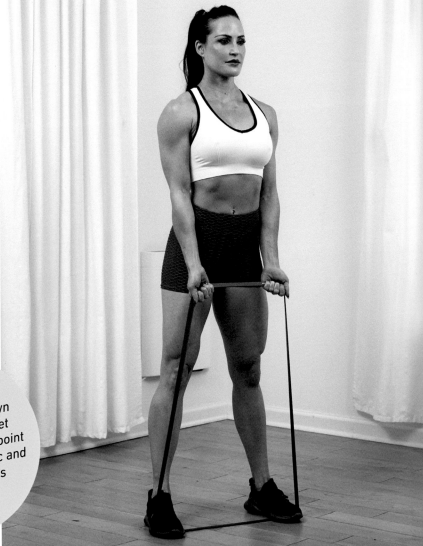

///// **TIP** /////
Focus on slowing down your tempo as you get closer to the mid-rep point on both the concentric and eccentric portions of the rep.

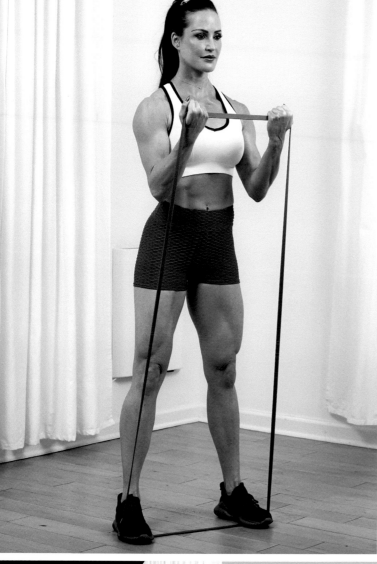

[2] Keeping your upper arms still, your shoulders back, and your wrists straight, slowly pull the band up toward your chest by contracting your biceps and flexing your elbows. Pause briefly just before your forearm reaches perpendicular to the floor.

[3] Slowly lower the band back down to a point just above the starting position to maintain tension in the band.

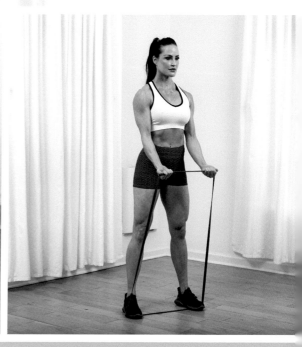

VARIATIONS

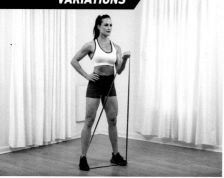

SINGLE-ARM BANDED BICEPS CURL Secure the band as instructed and perform the exercise using one arm at a time. Switch sides and perform the same number of reps on the opposite arm. (Make sure the tension is even on both sides.)

HIGH BICEPS CURL Attach a resistance band to a doorframe or other sturdy object at about chest height. Grasp the band with an underhand grip, extend your arms out in front of you, and then back away to create tension. Slowly pull the band upward and toward the top of your head, keeping your upper arm parallel to the floor throughout the exercise.

TARGETS /// **biceps (primary); none (secondary)**
EQUIPMENT /// **bench, dumbbells**

SPIDER CURL

If you have dominant shoulders and traps, this biceps curl variation is for you. And by performing the biceps curl on an incline, you'll be able to better isolate the biceps and take more dominant muscle groups out of the picture. You'll also eliminate momentum from the exercise, which can greatly improve results. The result will be beautifully peaked biceps and a more balanced upper body.

TRAIN THE RIGHT WAY

DO: Work on maintaining tension on the biceps by not allowing your forearms to reach perpendicular to the floor at any point.

DON'T: Allow your shoulders to round.

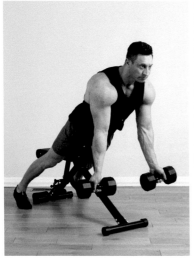

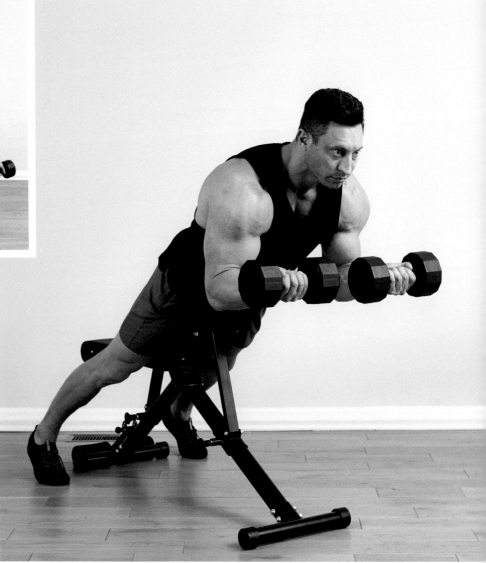

[1] Adjust the bench to a 60-degree angle. Lie stomach down on the bench with your legs straight and toes on the floor. Hold the dumbbells using an underhand grip with your arms extended toward the floor.

[2] Using only your elbows as hinges, pull the dumbbells upward using just your biceps.

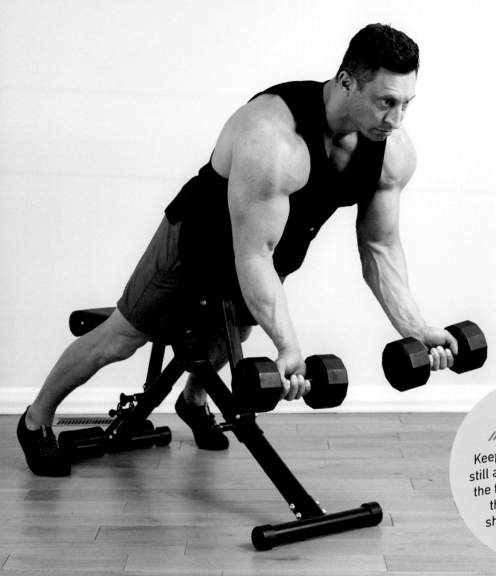

[3] Pause slightly when you feel your biceps fully contract, and then slowly lower the dumbbells back down to a point just short of the starting position to keep tension in the muscles.

///// **TIP** /////

Keep your upper arms still and perpendicular to the floor as you perform the exercise to limit shoulder contribution.

VARIATIONS

❮ **ALTERNATING ARM SPIDER CURL (MORE CHALLENGING)** Perform the exercise using one arm at a time while alternating back and forth between arms. Keep the nonworking arm at the mid-rep point instead of keeping it fully extended. (This variation increases the difficulty and can improve muscle contraction.)

CONCENTRATION CURL Stand facing the high end of an incline bench. Grasp a dumbbell in one hand, and place your working arm over the top end of the bench. With your elbow-in line with your shoulder, slowly curl the dumbbell up toward you. Repeat on the opposite side. (This variation is excellent for hitting the biceps peak.)

TARGETS /// **triceps (primary); forearms (secondary)**
EQUIPMENT /// **dumbbells, bench**

DUMBBELL SKULLCRUSHER

Despite its hardcore name, the skullcrusher is one of the most effective exercises for targeting the triceps. Using dumbbells means you must exert even effort to move the dumbbells in unison. Though the standard movement focuses on the long head of the triceps, you can hit all three heads by changing your grip, the angle of the bench, or the angle of your upper arm.

TRAIN THE RIGHT WAY

DO: Keep your upper arms fixed and just short of perpendicular to the floor.

DON'T: Go too heavy as other muscles will take over. (It can also be dangerous.)

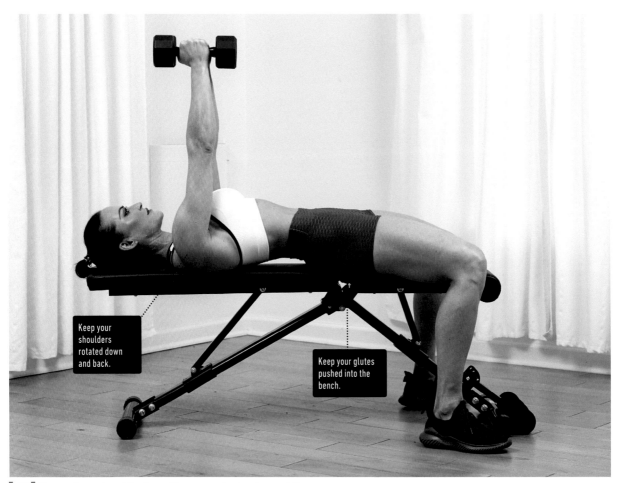

Keep your shoulders rotated down and back.

Keep your glutes pushed into the bench.

[1] Grasp two dumbbells with an neutral grip and lie on a flat bench with your feet flat on the floor. Extend the dumbbells overhead, allowing the dumbbells to touch.

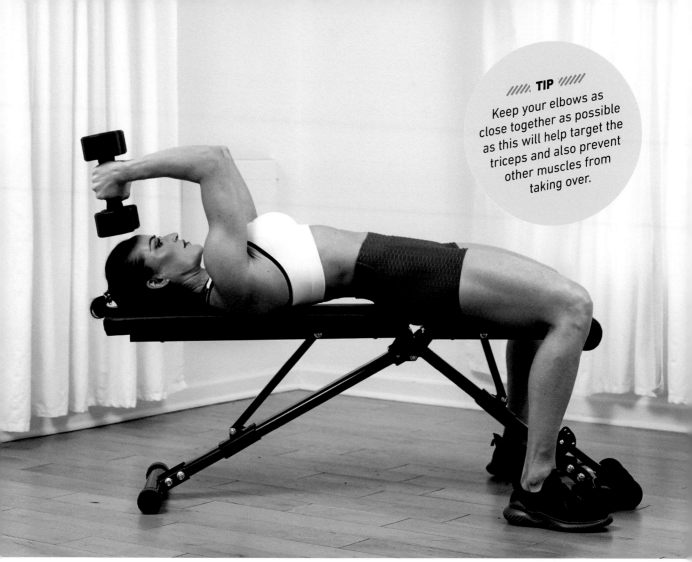

//// TIP ////

Keep your elbows as close together as possible as this will help target the triceps and also prevent other muscles from taking over.

[2] Keeping your upper arms fixed, lower the dumbbells down toward your forehead, using your elbows as a hinge. Pause about 1 inch (2.5cm) from your forehead, and then push the dumbbells back up to the starting position.

VARIATIONS

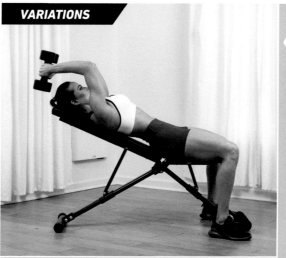

INCLINE BENCH SKULLCRUSHER (MORE CHALLENGING) Set the bench to a 45-degree angle. Fix your upper arms close to perpendicular to the floor, or a little beyond. Extend through the elbow as you would with the standard skullcrusher.

SINGLE-ARM SKULLCRUSHER Perform the exercise one arm at a time using only one dumbbell. (This variation allows you to go heavier since you will be self-spotting with the nonworking arm.)

TARGETS /// **triceps (primary); chest, lats (secondary)**
EQUIPMENT /// **resistance band**

BANDED TRICEPS PUSH-DOWN

Well-developed triceps not only add curves and shape to the arm, but they help balance capped delts. Use great care and discipline when performing this exercise as the triceps can be difficult to isolate without other muscle groups taking over. Focus on slowing down the tempo near the mid-rep point to improve the mind-muscle connection and to ensure you're isolating and working the triceps properly.

TRAIN THE RIGHT WAY

DO: Keep your upper body still and your shoulders back.

DON'T: Use momentum or lean forward excessively as both can cause other muscles to take over.

[1] Secure a resistance band to a door frame or a sturdy object at about forehead height. Grasp the ends of the band with an overhand grip and with your hands positioned about one hand width apart. Step away from the anchor point to create tension in the band, and then hinge at the hips to lean forward to about a 30-degree angle.

///// **TIP** /////
Keep constant tension on the band throughout the exercise.

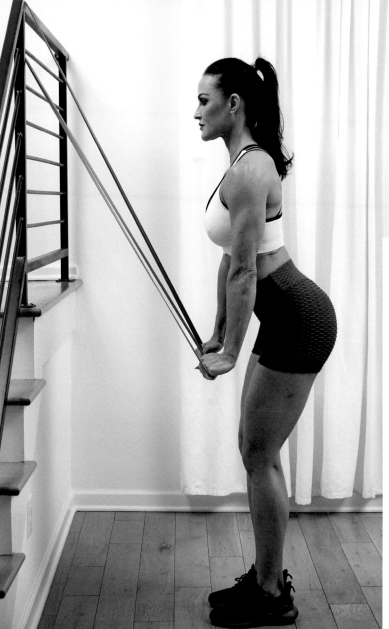

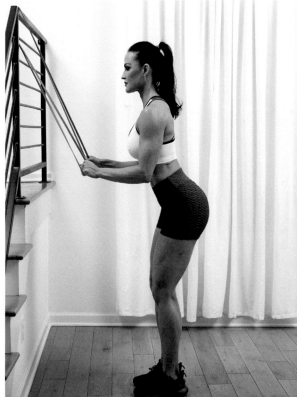

[2] With your upper arms held close to your body and your elbows pinned at your sides, push the band downward until your arms are fully extended.

[3] Slowly control the band back to a point just before the starting position to keep tension in the band.

VARIATIONS

SINGLE-ARM TRICEPS PUSH-DOWN Grasp the band with an overhand grip, and get into the starting position as instructed. Perform the exercise one arm at a time, preferably starting with the nondominant arm first, and then letting that arm dictate the number of reps you do on the dominant side.

WIDE-GRIP TRICEPS PUSH-DOWN Grasp the band with an overhand grip, and separate your hands to about shoulder width. Perform the exercise as instructed, maintaining the same width between your hands throughout the exercise. (Experiment with different grip widths and hand positions to target different areas of the triceps—wider grips tend to focus on the long and medial heads of the triceps.)

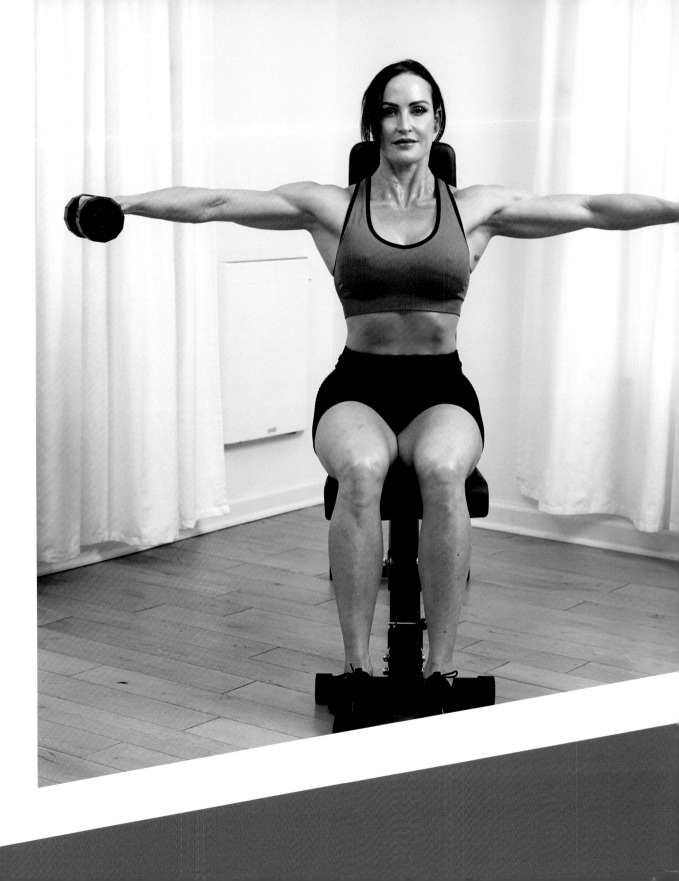

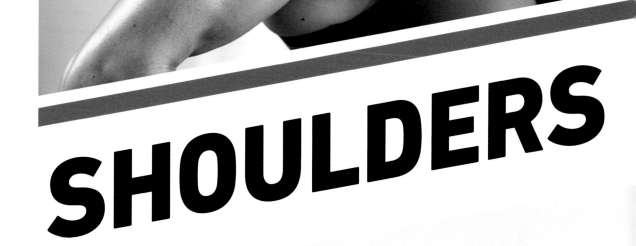

SHOULDERS

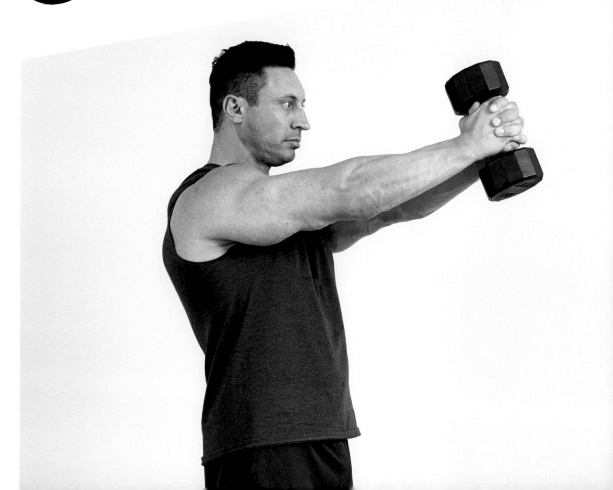

TARGETS /// **delts, chest (primary); triceps, core (secondary)**
EQUIPMENT /// **bench, dumbbells**

SEATED SHOULDER PRESS

The shoulder press is a variation of one of the six basic lifts. Master it and you'll build broad, strong shoulders and a tighter core, and also increase your overall power. In addition to enjoying the strength and aesthetic benefits, you'll be able to incorporate countless variations to better target any part of the delts once you become proficient in this basic lift.

TRAIN THE RIGHT WAY

DO: Go lighter on this exercise until you build up enough strength and stability to go heavier.

DON'T: Push your head forward at full extension. Your body should come forward.

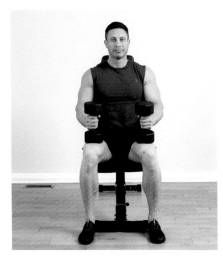

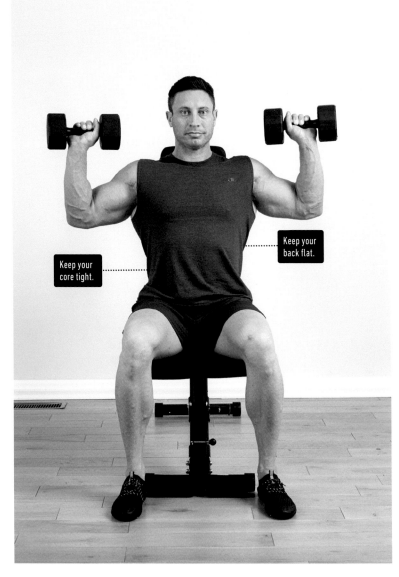

Keep your core tight.

Keep your back flat.

[1] Adjust the bench so the back is perpendicular to the floor. (Alternatively, you can set the bench flat and perform the exercise without back support.) Grasp the dumbbells and place them on their ends on top of your quads and just above your knees.

[2] Get into the starting position by using your legs to "kick" the dumbbells up so they're at about shoulder level, parallel to the floor, and about shoulder width apart. Keep your wrists straight and your elbows directly under your hands. Sit back against the bench.

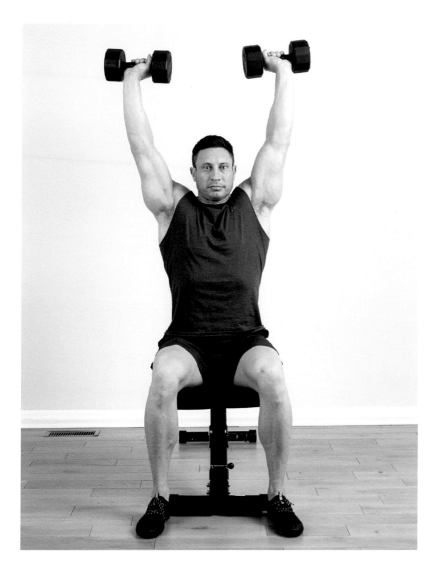

[3] Push the dumbbells upward until your arms are fully extended and in-line with your ears at full extension. Slowly lower the dumbbells back down while rotating your shoulder blades back and down as you come back to the starting position. (You should end the rep with your upper arms at or just below parallel to the floor.)

//// **TIP** ////

Always lock your shoulder blades back and down while pressing. (This will improve shoulder strength and also maintain shoulder health.)

VARIATIONS

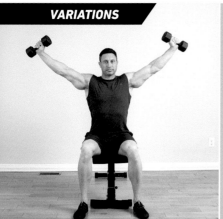

Y-PRESS Choose dumbbells that are 50 to 60 percent of the weight you would normally use. Start with an overhand grip, and hold the dumbbells at shoulder width. As you press, simultaneously push the dumbbells upward and outward into the shape of a *Y*.

PIKE PRESS (MORE CHALLENGING) Place your feet and hands flat on the floor with your hands positioned just wider than shoulder width. Straighten your legs to push your glutes upward until your upper body is close to perpendicular to the floor when your arms are fully extended. Slowly lower your upper body down until your upper arms are close to parallel to the floor. Using your delts, press yourself back up to the starting position.

BANDED SHOULDER PRESS (MORE CHALLENGING) Secure a resistance band under the bench, ensuring that it's secured directly in the middle of the band. Grasp the ends and perform the press as you would with dumbbells. (This variation can be done with just a band, or you can perform it with both dumbbells and a band to increase resistance and difficulty.)

TARGETS /// **delts, traps (primary); forearms (secondary)**
EQUIPMENT /// **dumbbells**

WIDE-GRIP UPRIGHT ROW

The upright row is traditionally performed with a bar and a more narrow grip. This variation uses a wider grip and dumbbells, which not only makes it better for at-home training but can make it more comfortable for your wrists and shoulders. The upright row adds width and dimension to your side and rear delts to create the look of a smaller waist and that classic X-frame shape.

TRAIN THE RIGHT WAY

DO: Keep your shoulder blades back and down to limit the use of the traps.

DON'T: Allow your wrists to bend. (This will help to maintain wrist health.)

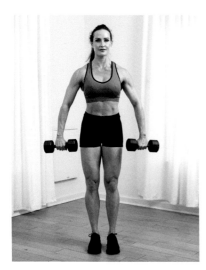

[1] Grasp the dumbbells with an overhand grip and stand with your feet shoulder width apart. Hold the dumbbells with your arms extended down and out at a point that is about twice as wide as your shoulders.

[2] Slowly pull the dumbbells upward, focusing on using just the delts as you pull. Pause momentarily when your upper arms reach parallel to the floor or just before your wrists begin to flex.

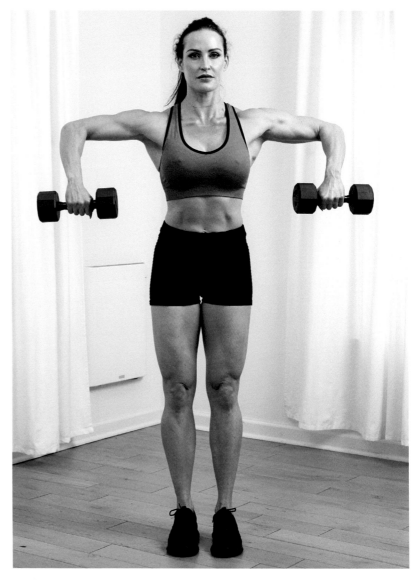

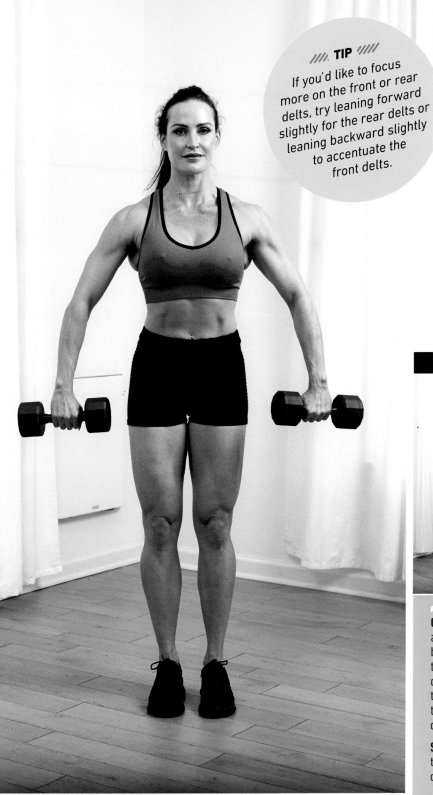

TIP

If you'd like to focus more on the front or rear delts, try leaning forward slightly for the rear delts or leaning backward slightly to accentuate the front delts.

[3] Slowly lower the dumbbells back down to the starting position, stopping just before your arms are fully extended.

VARIATIONS

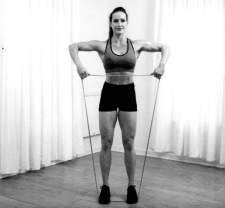

▲ BANDED UPRIGHT ROW (MORE CHALLENGING) Stand in the middle of a looped resistance band, and hold the band with an overhand grip. Perform the upright row as you would with dumbbells. (Depending on the band tension, you may want to shorten the range of motion to keep tension on the delts.)

SINGLE-ARM UPRIGHT ROW Perform the exercise as instructed, using only one arm at a time.

TARGETS /// **rear delts, rhomboids (primary); lats, traps (secondary)**
EQUIPMENT /// **dumbbell**

DUMBBELL FACE PULL

With a light dumbbell and a precise range of motion, you can target the rear delts with this exercise that is typically done on a cable machine. The rear delts, though small, make a big impact on your silhouette by adding width and definition to the back of the shoulders. This not only ties the shoulders in nicely with the back but also helps to accentuate the v-taper.

TRAIN THE RIGHT WAY

DO: Keep constant tension on the rear delts once you feel them engage by stopping just before your arms are fully extended at the end of the rep.

DON'T: Use a dumbbell that's too heavy, which can cause your traps and lats to take over.

[1] Grasp each end of a light dumbbell with an overhand grip. Stand with your feet shoulder width apart, and then bend forward at the hips until your upper body is just above parallel to the floor. Extend your arms downward so they're just in-line with your chin.

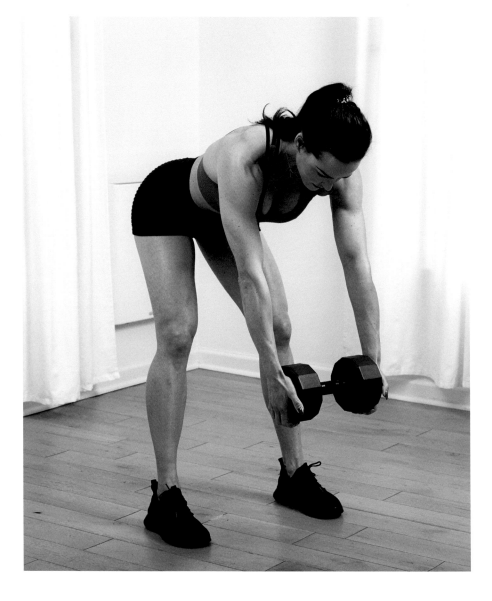

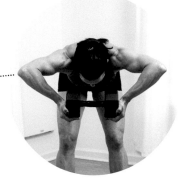

Keep your elbows out.

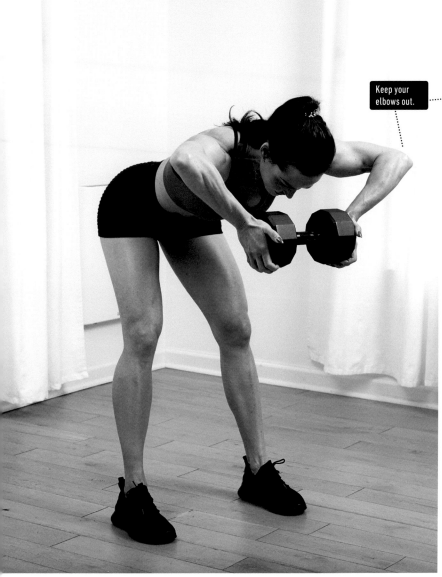

[2] Slowly pull the dumbbell up toward your chin, allowing your elbows to flare outward as you pull. Pause momentarily as your hands approach your face, and then slowly lower the dumbbell back down to the starting position, pausing just before your arms are fully extended.

/// **TIP** ///

Think about keeping your elbows up throughout the exercise to limit the use of the lats.

VARIATIONS

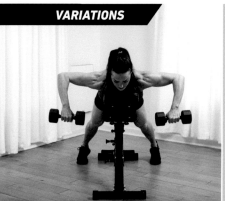

INCLINE BENCH UPRIGHT ROW Set the bench to about 70 degrees. Lay stomach down on the bench. Using light dumbbells and keeping your elbows high, legs straight, and toes on the floor, pull the dumbbells straight up. (Try not to let yourself rest at the bottom of the exercise so you can keep constant tension on the muscle.)

BANDED FACE PULL Secure a band around a sturdy object at about chin height. With an overhand grip, slowly pull the band toward your nose, keeping your elbows high throughout the range of motion. (Limit the range of motion to keep constant tension in the band.)

SINGLE-ARM BANDED FACE PULL Secure the band as you would with the banded face pull variation, but perform the exercise using only one arm at a time.

TARGETS /// **front and medial delts (primary); triceps, core (secondary)**
EQUIPMENT /// **dumbbell**

DUMBBELL PRESS-OUT

A unique exercise, the dumbbell press-out can give you that last little push needed to grow your shoulders. This exercise is a hybrid between a thruster and a shoulder press and is well suited as either a workout finisher or as an initial exercise to get your heart rate up. Start with a lighter dumbbell as fatigue can set in quickly.

TRAIN THE RIGHT WAY

DO: Keep the rest of your body still, and focus on using only your shoulders.

DON'T: Go too heavy as this exercise can be more difficult than it looks.

[1] Using an interlocking grip, grasp a dumbbell with the end facing up. (Your knuckles should be facing out.) Stand with your feet shoulder width apart and with soft knees. Begin with the top of the dumbbell positioned just under your collarbone

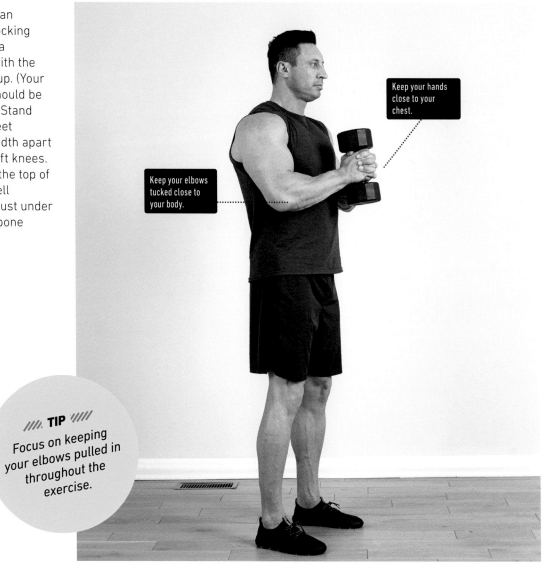

Keep your hands close to your chest.

Keep your elbows tucked close to your body.

//// TIP ////
Focus on keeping your elbows pulled in throughout the exercise.

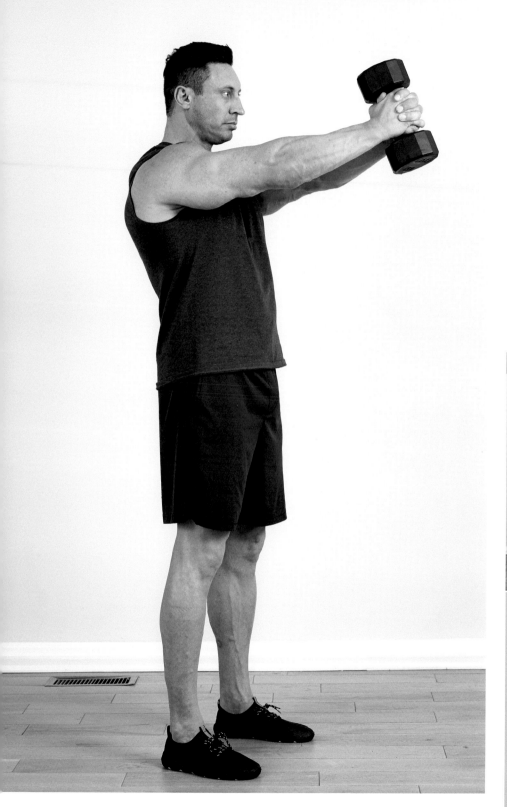

[2] Press the dumbbell slightly upward and outward, keeping your elbows lower than the dumbbell as you press. Press to a full arm extension, and then slowly pull the dumbbell back to the starting position.

VARIATIONS

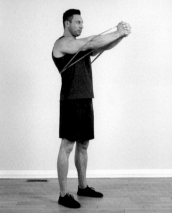

▲ BANDED PRESS-OUT
Loop a resistance band around your lower-mid back. Grasp the ends, interlock your fingers, and perform the exercise as you would if using a dumbbell.

SINGLE-ARM PRESS-OUT
Hold a lighter dumbbell with a neutral grip and perform the exercise using one arm at a time.

TARGETS /// **side delts (primary); forearms (secondary)**
EQUIPMENT /// **bench, dumbbells**

LATERAL RAISE

When trained effectively, the medial delts can add width across the upper body, which can create the illusion of a smaller waist. Choose a weight that's on the lighter side to start, and focus on the cue of "pushing" the dumbbells away from you instead of lifting the dumbbells up. This can keep the traps and other surrounding muscles from contributing to the effort.

TRAIN THE RIGHT WAY

DO: Maintain a slight bend in the elbows throughout the move, and keep the rest of your body still.

DON'T: Bounce with each rep.

[1] Sit on the bench at a 90-degree angle with your upper body tall and your feet flat on the floor. Hold the dumbbells at your sides, using an overhand grip with your palms facing down. Bend your arms just slightly.

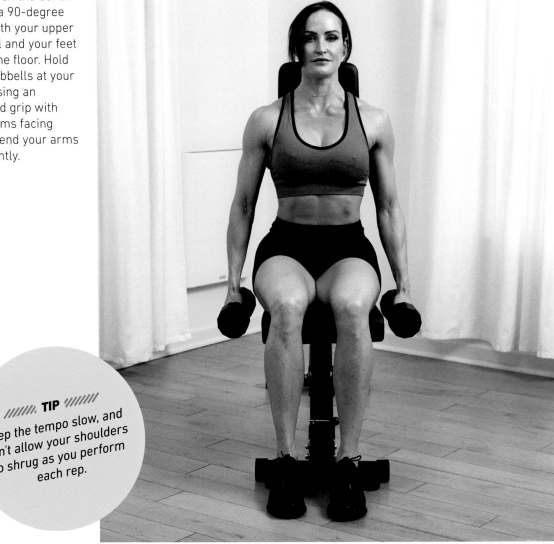

///// **TIP** /////
Keep the tempo slow, and don't allow your shoulders to shrug as you perform each rep.

[2] Raise the dumbbells in an arc, keeping your arms extended with just a slight bend. Pause slightly when your upper arms reach just above parallel to the floor.

[3] Control the weight back down to a point just above the starting point.

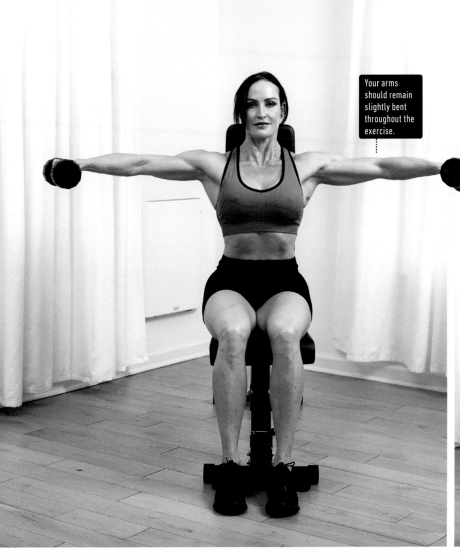

Your arms should remain slightly bent throughout the exercise.

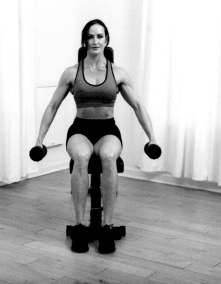

VARIATIONS

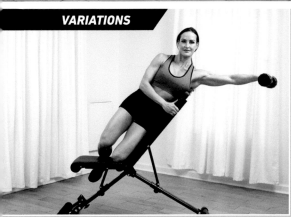

▶ **INCLINE BENCH 45-DEGREE LATERAL RAISE** Adjust your bench to 45 degrees, and carefully lie on your side with your bottom arm draped over the top of the bench and your bottom hand holding a dumbbell. Perform all of the reps on one side, and then switch to the opposite side. (Incline bench 45-degree lateral raises can isolate the delts and keep the traps from contributing to the movement.)

BANDED LATERAL RAISE (MORE CHALLENGING) While standing, hold light dumbbells and a light resistance band. Step on the middle of the resistance band. Perform the exercise as instructed. (This variation adds resistance at the midpoint of the rep.)

TARGETS /// **medial and rear delts, rhomboids, traps (primary);**
upper lats (secondary)
EQUIPMENT /// **bench, dumbbells**

REVERSE FLYE

The front delts tend to get worked when training the chest and arms. This can cause the delts to look out of balance as the front of the shoulder can become more developed than the side and rear. The solution is to carefully choose exercises to "bring up" the medial and rear delts. The result is beautifully capped shoulders that create impressive width across the upper body. Choose lighter weights when performing this exercise to ensure that the stronger lats or traps don't take over.

TRAIN THE RIGHT WAY

DO: Think about pushing the dumbbells away from each other versus pulling them upward. This can help keep the traps from engaging.

DON'T: Go too heavy as other muscle groups can take over.

[**1**] Adjust your bench to a 60-degree angle. Grasp a light set of dumbbells, and lie stomach down on the bench with your legs extended, your toes on the floor, and your chest flat on the bench. Extend your arms downward, with your palms facing each other.

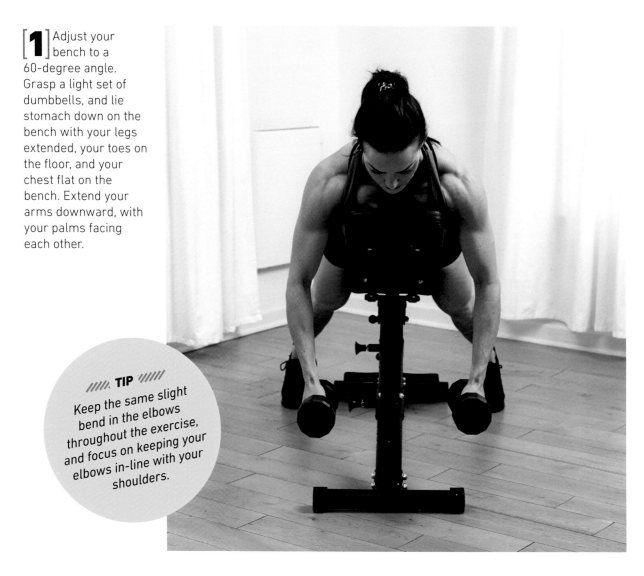

///// **TIP** /////
Keep the same slight bend in the elbows throughout the exercise, and focus on keeping your elbows in-line with your shoulders.

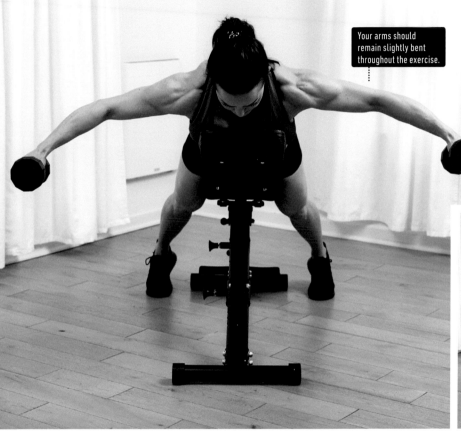

[2] With a soft bend in the elbows, slowly raise the dumbbells upward and outward in an arc that stops at about chin height.

[3] Slowly lower the dumbbells back down to a point just above the starting position to keep constant tension on the muscles.

Your arms should remain slightly bent throughout the exercise.

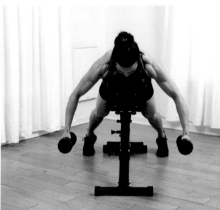

VARIATIONS

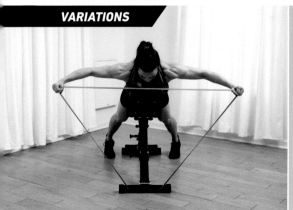

BANDED REVERSE FLYE Secure a resistance band under the front foot of the bench. Grasp the band using a neutral grip and perform the exercise as you would with dumbbells. (Be sure to keep constant tension on the delts.)

BAND PULL APART Grasp a resistance band with both hands using an overhand grip. Stand with your feet shoulder width apart and extend your arms outward. Slowly pull your hands apart, making sure to have tension on the band from the starting position. Pull horizontally until you feel strong tension and then return to the starting position. (The range of motion will be between 12 and 18 inches in total).

TARGETS /// **front and medial delts delts (primary); traps, chest (secondary)**
EQUIPMENT /// **dumbbell**

BUS DRIVER

When training at home, a little creativity goes a long way. If you have never tried bus drivers, get ready for a tougher-than-it-looks exercise and a great pump. As an added benefit, this exercise strengthens the rotator cuffs to help avoid common injuries to this area. Though commonly performed using a weight plate, a dumbbell works just as well for this exercise.

[**1**] Stand with your feet shoulder width apart and your knees soft. With a tight core, grasp each end of a dumbbell, and extend your arms straight out in front of you.

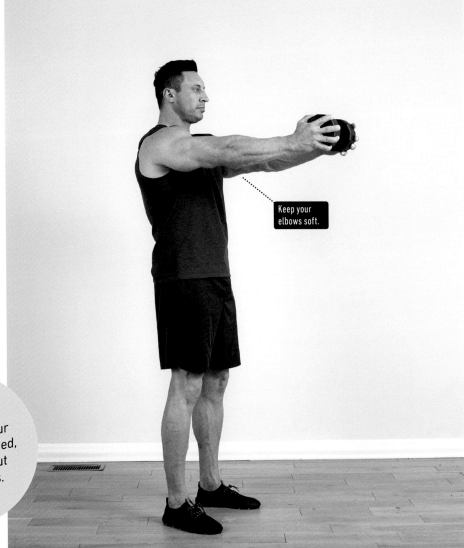

Keep your elbows soft.

/// TIP ////
Even though your arms are extended, do not lock out your elbows.

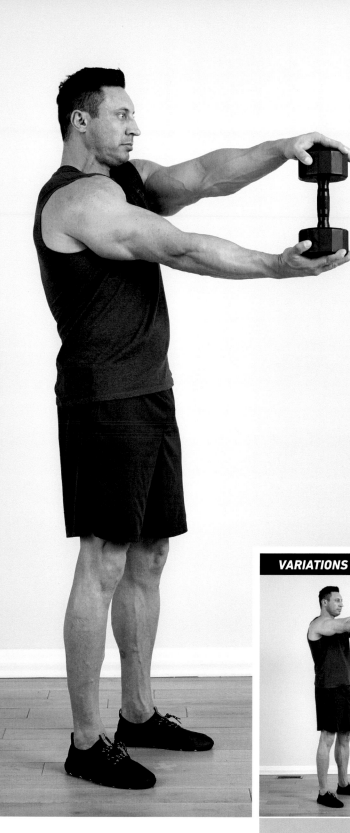

[2] Keeping your arms extended, slowly rotate the dumbbell until it is perpendicular to the floor. (Think of turning a steering wheel.)

[3] Pause slightly, and then slowly rotate the dumbbell in the opposite direction until you reach perpendicular.

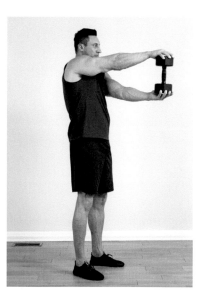

VARIATIONS

‹ SINGLE DUMBBELL FRONT RAISE Holding each end of a dumbbell, extend your arms straight out. Slowly lower your arms to almost perpendicular to the floor, and then lift the dumbbell back to the starting position.

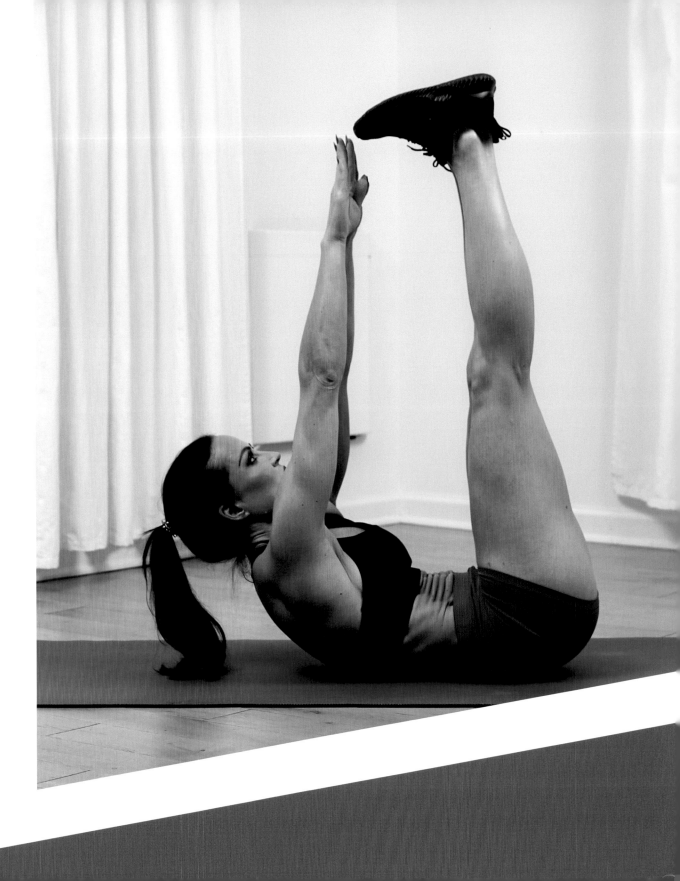

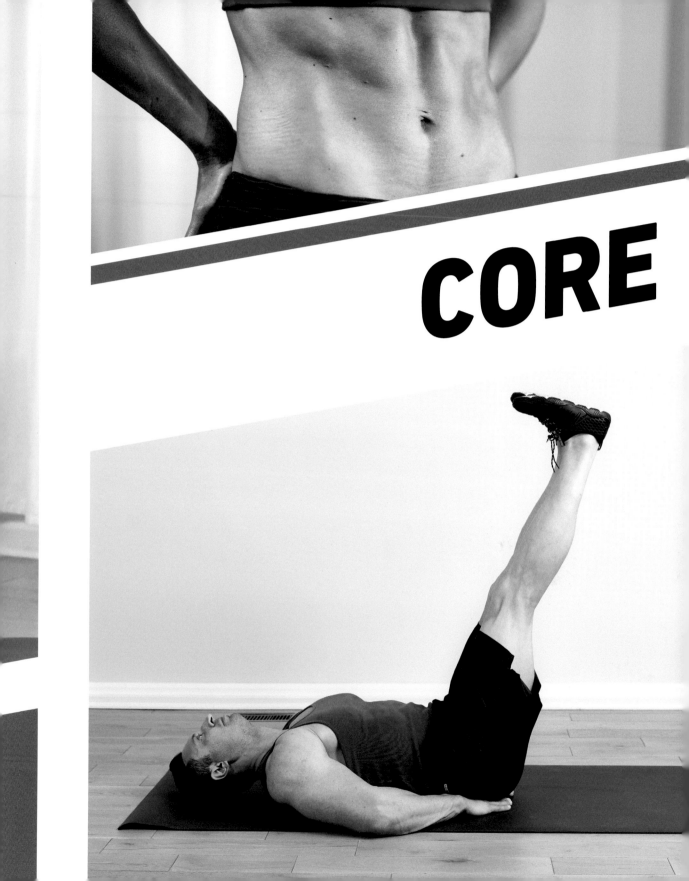

CORE

TARGETS /// **transverse abdominis (TVA), abs, lower back (primary); shoulders, quads (secondary)**

EQUIPMENT /// **yoga mat or towel**

X PLANK

If your goal is to shape a smaller waist and gain definition, planks and their variations can help you achieve those goals. The X plank is a tougher variation of the basic plank and targets the abdominal muscles you can't see (or the transverse abdominis [TVA]). Trimming size from your waist and strengthening your core can help prevent injury and make all of your compound lifts stronger.

TRAIN THE RIGHT WAY

DO: Focus on keeping your hips in-line with your shoulders and keeping your spine neutral to help keep the rest of your body in-line.

DON'T: Look up or let your hips drop or rise above your shoulders.

[**1**] Lie stomach down on the floor, and then rise up into a high plank position with your arms extended straight down.

[**2**] Slowly walk your hands outward and upward until your arms form a V shape. Step your feet outward to form a wider base. (Your body should resemble an X shape.) Hold for as long as you can.

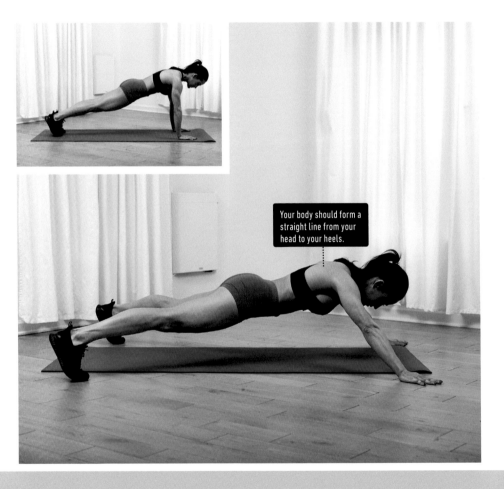

Your body should form a straight line from your head to your heels.

VARIATIONS

HIGH-SIDE PLANK Perform the exercise while on your side with your working arm extended straight down and your hand flat on the floor. (Your weight will rest on the side of one foot.) Your body should be in a straight line from the ground up and from head to toes. Repeat on the opposite side.

HIGH PLANK LEG LIFT Get into high plank position and alternate lifting each leg upward while focusing on contracting the glute and keeping the leg straight while lifting. (This variation hits the glutes and core.)

TARGETS /// transverse abdominis (TVA), abs (primary); obliques (secondary)
EQUIPMENT /// yoga mat or towel

VACUUM

With so much fuss around waist training, many have taken to wearing corsets in an attempt to decrease waist size. The results of this are temporary, and waist training itself can cause unhealthy side effects. A better and more lasting option is the vacuum. Classic era bodybuilders were known for their incredible small waists and would practice vacuums a few times per week. Take the time to perfect the vacuum, and you'll not only enjoy a smaller waist but you'll also increase your core strength.

TRAIN THE RIGHT WAY:

DO: Try to perform vacuums on an empty stomach and first thing in the morning.

DON'T: Let your inability to hold your breath for longer periods of time stop you—it's okay to take small, shallow breaths as needed.

[**1**] Kneel on the floor with your back slightly rounded and your hands on your knees.

[**2**] Slowly expell all the air from your lungs, and hold your breath as you focus on pulling your belly button up toward your ribcage. (This should feel like you're taking a deep breath. Think about closing your windpipe, expanding your ribcage, and pulling your diaphragm inward.) Hold the pose for as long as you can, slowly building up the hold time as you improve your endurance and mind-muscle control.

VARIATIONS

LYING VACUUM (EASIER) Lie down with your back flat on the floor and your pelvis rolled forward. Perform the exercise as instructed.

PULL-DOWN VACUUM CRUNCH (MORE CHALLENGING) Secure a band at the top of a door frame. Grasp the band with both hands and kneel to the floor. Perform the vacuum, using the band for resistance as you simultaneously do a crunch while holding the vacuum. (This variation further strengthens the TVA, in addition to the rectus abdominis, also known as the "six-pack.")

TARGETS /// **rectus abdominis (primary); obliques (secondary)**
EQUIPMENT /// **resistance band, yoga mat**

BANDED CRUNCH

If you've performed standard crunches before, you know the exercise can become monotonous and also ineffective unless you continue to add reps. This crunch variation adds a resistance band to increase the difficulty, especially at the mid-rep point of the exercise. By using a resistance band, you'll also able to get away with fewer reps than you would with traditional bodyweight crunches.

TRAIN THE RIGHT WAY

DO: Try to keep your arms, neck, and lower body locked into place.

DON'T: Tuck your chin or pull on your head as you crunch. (This can cause injury.)

[**1**] Anchor a resistance band over the top of a door or other sturdy overhead anchor point. Grasp the ends of the resistance band with an underhand grip and lower yourself into a kneeling position while facing away from the anchor point. Hold the band with your palms facing your traps and your hands resting on your traps. Lean forward to create tension in the band.

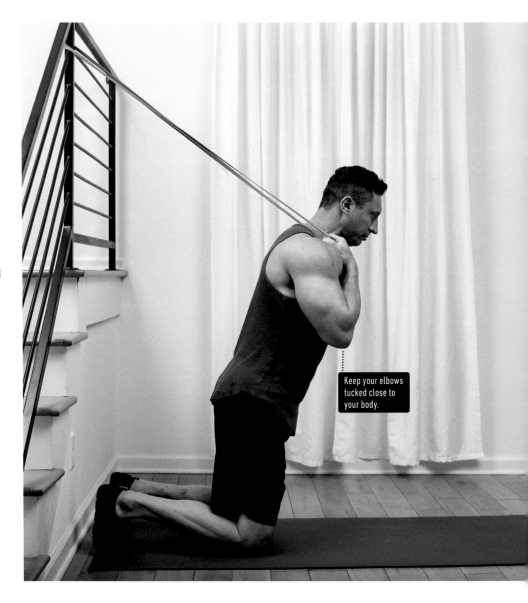

Keep your elbows tucked close to your body.

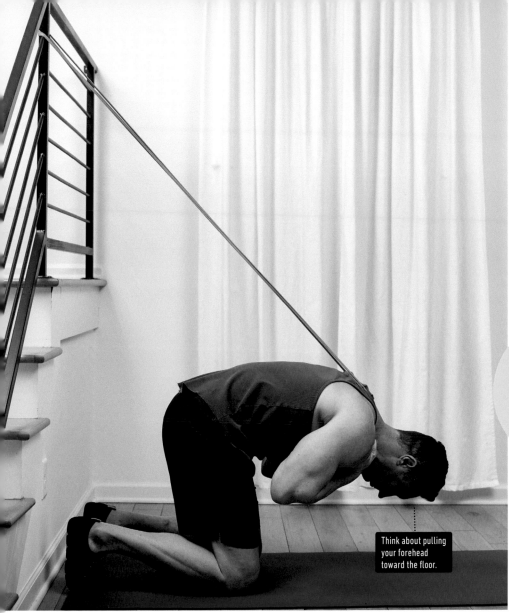

[2] Slowly pull your upper body downward, engaging your abs as you pull. (Allow your back to round slightly as this will help engage the abs.) Pause momentarily when your head reaches close to hip level, and then slowly return to the starting position.

TIP

Exhale as you crunch. This will help you contract the abs more effectively.

Think about pulling your forehead toward the floor.

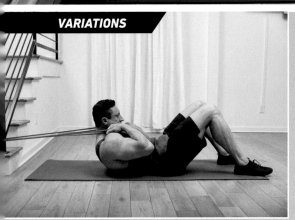

BANDED CURL-UP Attach a resistance band to a sturdy object at about shin height. Lie flat, facing away from the anchor point, and grasp the ends of the bands, pulling them close to your traps. Tuck your elbows in close to your body, and lock them into place. Keeping your upper back slightly rounded, engage your core and pull your chin toward your knees, and then control your upper body back to the starting position.

REVERSE BAND CRUNCH Attach the resistance band to a door at about knee height. Sit on the floor, facing the band, and loop the band around your legs. Lie back on the floor and place your hands under your hips. Slowly pull your legs upward and toward your upper body. (As you pull, your hips will lift off the floor.) Pause momentarily, and then return to the starting position.

TARGETS /// **obliques, abs (primary); hip flexors (secondary)**
EQUIPMENT /// **yoga mat or towel**

KNEE-UP

Knee-ups will strengthen your core, improve your balance, and target every muscle in the abs, including the rectus abdominis (or "six-pack"), along with your TVA, which acts as an internal girdle. This can also help with posture as you'll elongate your spine to assist in balancing your body. This is an advanced move, but you can make it easier by placing your hands on the floor to help with balance.

TRAIN THE RIGHT WAY

DO: Keep your core tight, and try not to engage your hip flexors.

DON'T: Round your shoulders or back.

[1] Sit on a yoga mat with your feet flat on the floor. Bring your knees up toward your chest as you extend your upper body to bring your chest up toward your knees. Bring both your feet and your hands off the floor as you slowly balance on your tailbone.

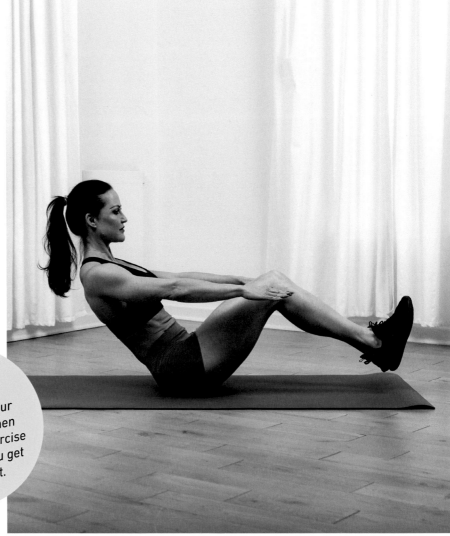

// **TIP** ///
Focus first on balancing on your tailbone, and then perform the exercise slowly until you get a feel for it.

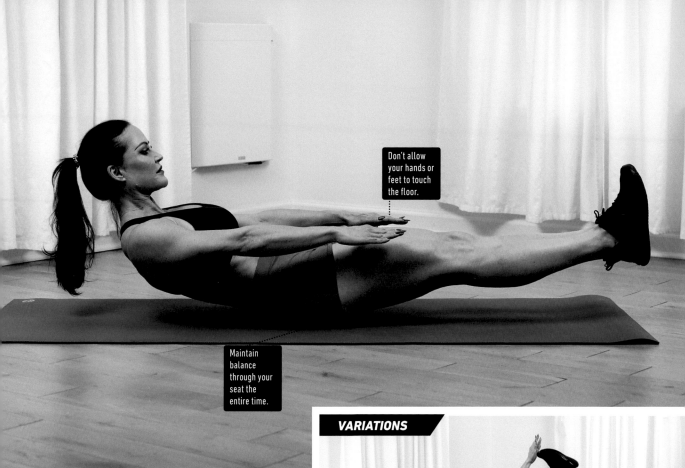

Don't allow your hands or feet to touch the floor.

Maintain balance through your seat the entire time.

[2] With your core engaged and back flat, simultaneously lower your upper and lower body to the floor, extending your legs as you lower down to a point just before you reach the floor. Engage your core to bring your upper body and lower body back up to the starting position.

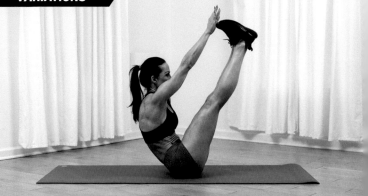

VARIATIONS

⌃ V-UP (MORE CHALLENGING) Rather than bending at the knees, extend your legs and arms straight. Simultaneously lift your upper and lower body off the floor. (Your body should resemble a *V* at the mid-rep point.)

BENCH KNEE-UP (EASIER) This variation is great for beginners. Rather than performing the exercise on the floor, sit across a bench. Hold onto the bench to help with balance, and then perform the exercise as instructed.

L-UP Lie back on the yoga mat, and tuck your hands under your hips. Extend your legs straight out, and raise them until they're perpendicular to the floor.

TARGETS /// **transverse abdominis (TVA), abs, (primary);**
hip flexors, lower back (secondary)
EQUIPMENT /// **yoga mat or towel**

HOLLOW HOLD

While this isometric exercise might look easy, it's a true test of core strength. It effectively strengthens all of the abdominal musculature, in addition to building lower-back strength. This move creates more strength for big compound movements, which can help you avoid injury. It also can create the appearance of a smaller waist.

TRAIN THE RIGHT WAY

DO: Keep your abs contracted, and push your lower back into the floor.

DON'T: Allow your lower back to come off the floor.

[1] Lie flat on your back on a yoga mat with your legs extended and your arms extended over your head.

[2] Push your lower back into the mat while slowly raising your upper body and legs off the floor until your head and shoulder blades are off the floor. Hold for the designated amount of time, focusing on contracting your abs and tucking your chin as you hold the pose, and then return to the starting position.

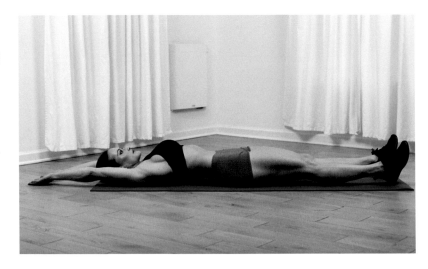

VARIATIONS

FLUTTER KICK Get into the hollow hold position. Slowly lower one leg downward and then bring it back up to the starting position. Repeat on the opposite side. (You can repeat this movement for reps or time.)

DEAD BUG From the hollow hold position, simultaneously lower one leg downward, while lowering the opposite arm to the floor. Bring your leg and arm back to the starting position, and then repeat on the opposite side. (You can repeat this movement for reps or time.)

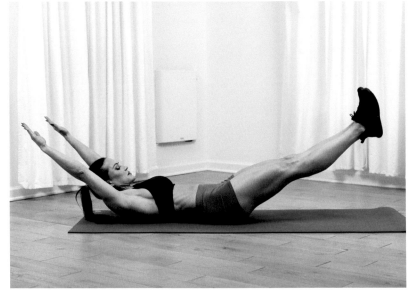

TARGETS /// **obliques, abs, transverse abdominis (TVA) (primary); hip flexors (secondary)**
EQUIPMENT /// **yoga mat or towel, mini band**

BANDED BICYCLE

Take the basic bicycle exercise to another level by incorporating a mini band. The increased tension will cause you to engage the abs more fully. And the band also acts as a form check—if you don't properly cycle your legs through, the band will go slack. As you perform this exercise, you'll be targeting and training all muscles in the abs, including the TVA. Over time, this move can help decrease waist circumference and also lead to a stronger core.

TRAIN THE RIGHT WAY

DO: Perform the exercise slowly until you're able to perfect the movement.

DON'T: Pull on your ears or head as you perform the exercise. (This can cause injury.)

[1] From a seated position, place the mini band around the arch of each foot. Lie back and extend your legs out in front of you. Lift your upper back and head off the floor, and make sure your lower back is pressed into the mat. Place your hands near your ears with your elbows out.

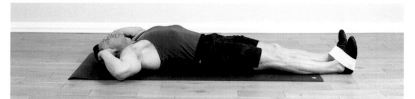

[2] Lift your legs off the floor slightly, keeping one leg fully extended, and then bring one knee toward your chest while bringing the opposite elbow forward until it almost touches the knee.

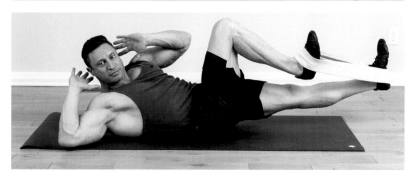

[3] Return the working arm and working leg to the starting position, and then bring the opposite knee and elbow up toward your midsection. Continue alternating sides until you reach the prescribed number of reps.

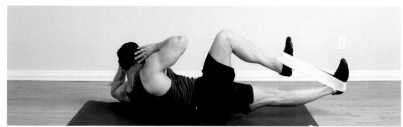

VARIATIONS

BANDED FLUTTER KICK Place the mini band around your ankles and lie flat on your back with your legs extended. Place your hands under your hips, and press your lower back into the floor as you lift both legs off the floor slightly. Lift one leg, keeping the other one still, then lower the lifted leg while lifting the other leg.

STANDING BICYCLE CRUNCH Stand with your feet shoulder-width apart. Place your hands near your ears with your elbows out. Raise one knee toward your chest and simultaneously lower your elbow to meet your knee, focusing on rounding your upper back and crunching your abs. Return your leg and elbow to the starting point and then repeat on the opposite sides.

TARGETS /// **obliques, lower back, transverse abdominis (TVA) (primary); shoulders, glutes (secondary)**
EQUIPMENT /// **yoga mat or towel**

SIDE PLANK

Traditional abs exercises tend to focus more on the rectus abdominis (or "six-pack"). Incorporating side planks into your routine will not only strengthen the obliques but also the lower back, which will improve overall core stability and lessen the risk of injury. Even though the side plank is classified as an abs exercise, you'll be working many other muscles in the body and also stabilizing with the shoulders, which will help create improved shoulder health.

TRAIN THE RIGHT WAY

DO: Keep your core engaged the entire time to help your body stay in alignment.

DON'T: Allow your hips to sag or raise them above the line of your body. (This can cause lower-back strain and make the exercise ineffective.)

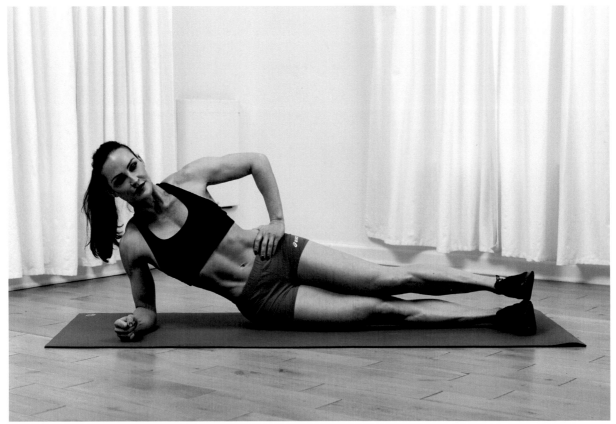

[1] Lie on a yoga mat and roll to one side, placing your elbow directly underneath your shoulder. With your legs extended, stack one leg on top of the other so that your body forms as straight a line as possible from your toes to your nose.

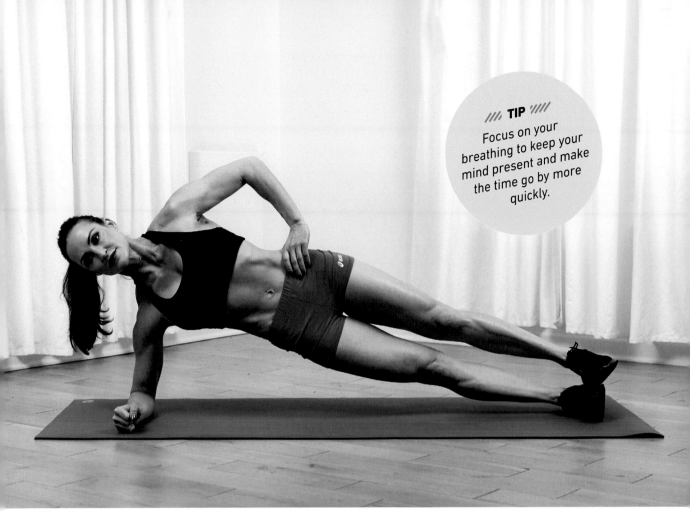

/// TIP ///
Focus on your breathing to keep your mind present and make the time go by more quickly.

[2] Lift your hip and upper leg off the mat until your body is in a straight diagonal line. Hold the pose for the designated amount of time, and then return to the starting position.

VARIATIONS

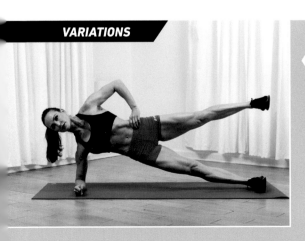

SIDE PLANK WITH ABDUCTOR LIFT Get into side plank position and then lift your top leg, keeping it fully extended until it reaches just above parallel to the floor.

SIDE PLANK ROW (MORE CHALLENGING) Attach a resistance band to a sturdy object just above floor height. Hold onto the band, and position your mat far enough away from the far end of the resistance band to create tension when your arm is extended and you're in the side plank position. Starting with your top arm extended, slowly pull the resistance band toward your body, keeping your elbow at your side. Pause briefly when your hand reaches your chest, and then extend your arm back to the starting point.

TARGETS /// **lower abs, obliques (primary); hip flexors (secondary)**
EQUIPMENT /// **yoga mat or towel**

TOE TOUCHER

Defined abs are created through a combination of building up the rectus abdominis (or "six-pack") and diet. Many abs exercises target the upper portion of the rectus abdominis, which are usually more readily visible as you get leaner, but the lower section of the six-pack can require more direct training to see results. Toe touchers are excellent for building up the lower abs and defining them.

TRAIN THE RIGHT WAY

DO: Control the speed of each rep and go slow, focusing on using just your abs.

DON'T: Allow your legs to move from perpendicular to the floor as this can cause lower-back strain.

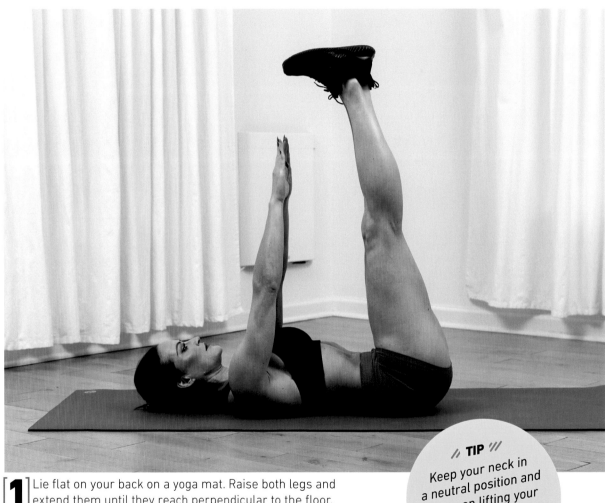

[1] Lie flat on your back on a yoga mat. Raise both legs and extend them until they reach perpendicular to the floor. Extend your arms up toward your feet.

// TIP //
Keep your neck in a neutral position and focus on lifting your upper body off the mat, using just your abs.

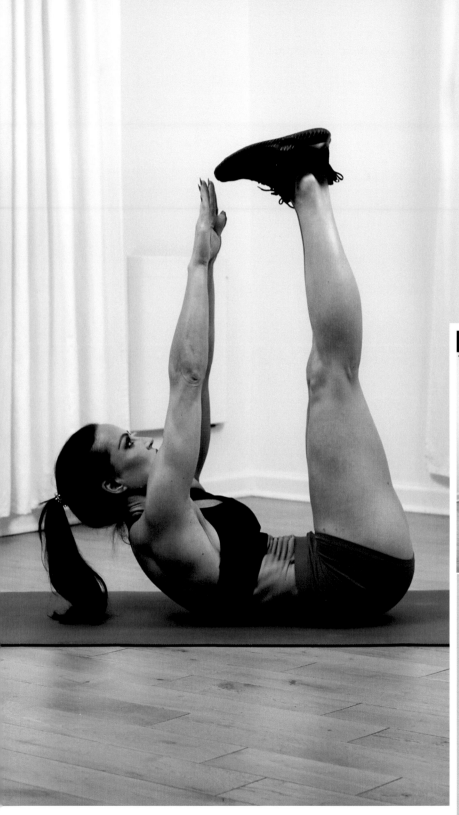

[2] Contract your abs, focusing on pushing your lower back into the mat and rounding your upper back to bring your shoulders up off the mat and your hands closer to your feet. Pause briefly when your shoulder blades are off the mat and your abs are fully contracted, and then return to the starting position.

VARIATIONS

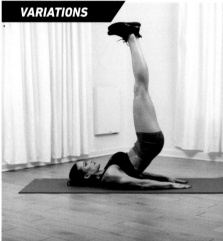

REVERSE CRUNCH Lie flat on the mat with your legs perpendicular to the floor. Place your hands under your hips for stability. Keeping your legs as straight as possible, contract your lower abs to bring your hips off the floor. Slowly lower your hips back down to the starting point.

REVERSE CRUNCH AGAINST A WALL (MORE CHALLENGING) Lie face up with your hips about 6 inches (15.25cm) from a wall and your legs parallel to the wall. Lift your hips off the floor, using the wall as a guide to keep your legs straight. (Don't rest your legs against the wall.)

TARGETS /// **abs, hip flexors, transverse abdominis (TVA) (primary); quads, lower back (secondary)**
EQUIPMENT /// **yoga mat or towel**

LYING LEG RAISE

Bodyweight exercises are a true test of strength, and the lying leg raise is no exception. In addition to targeting all abdominal muscles, it'll work your lower back and hip flexors. The leg raise is versatile, too, which allows you to mix things up with your training and continue making progress whenever one variation becomes too easy.

TRAIN THE RIGHT WAY

DO: Keep your lower back pressed into the mat and your head on the mat.

DON'T: Arch your back as this can add pressure on it.

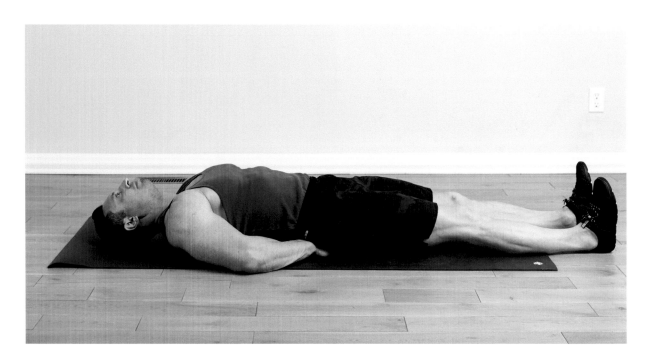

[1] Lie on your back with your hands tucked under your hips. Engage your core.

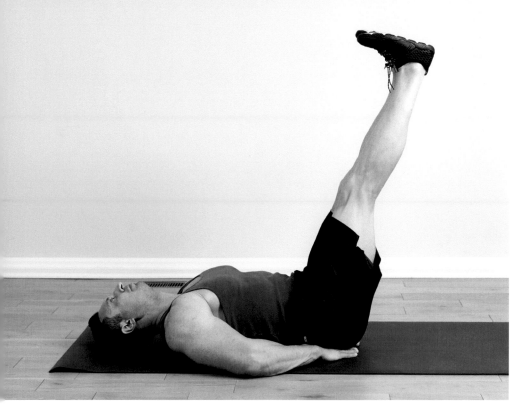

[2] Keeping your legs straight, lift them off the mat until they're almost perpendicular to the floor.

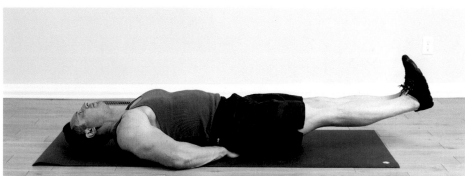

[3] Slowly lower your legs back down to a point just above floor height to keep tension in the muscles.

VARIATIONS

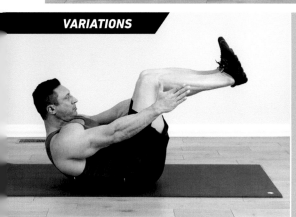

TUCK CRUNCH Lie on your back with your legs fully extended and your lower back pressed into the mat. Slowly pull your knees up to your chest while simultaneously lifting your shoulder blades off the mat and extending your arms upward and forward as you crunch. Return to the starting position and repeat.

ALTERNATING LYING LEG RAISE Begin the exercise as instructed, but instead of lifting both legs up, alternate by lifting one leg at a time.

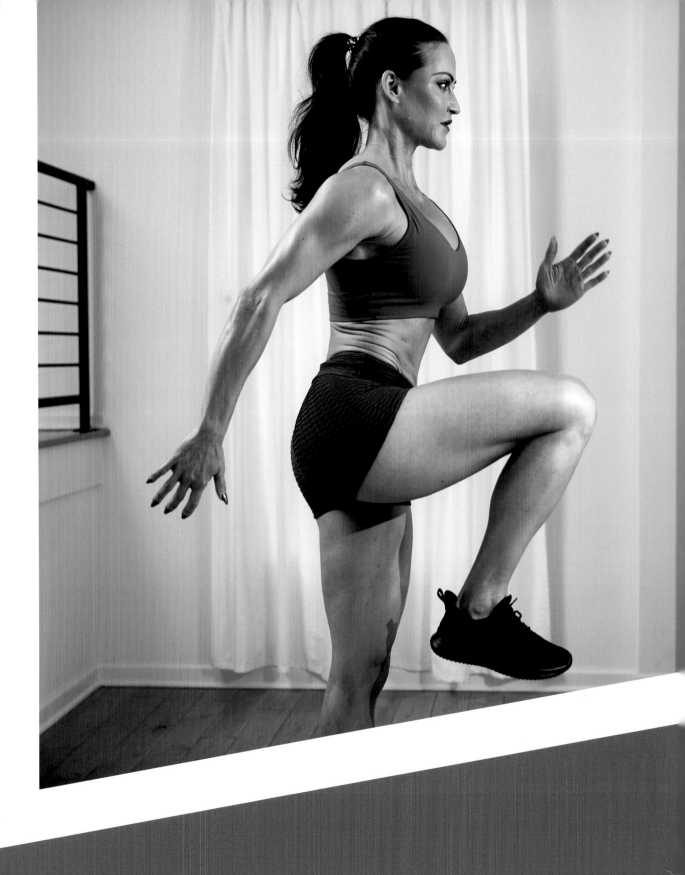

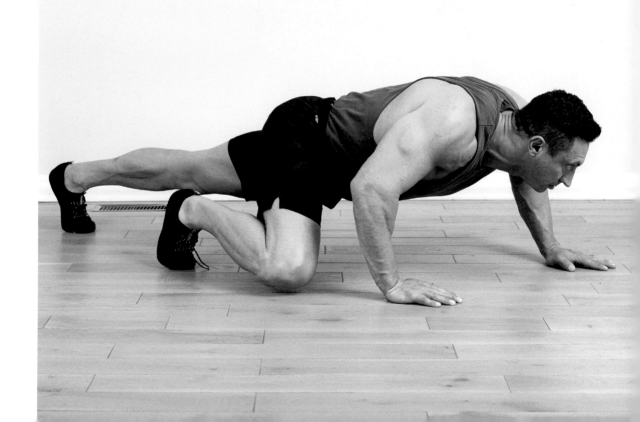

CARDIO

TARGETS /// **total body**
EQUIPMENT /// **none**

BURPEE

Build strength and endurance with this versatile, do-anywhere bodyweight exercise that can be modified to be easier or more difficult, allowing you to make progress over time. Burpees fit into almost any training program, whether you use them as a finisher, a standalone workout, or as part of a circuit. Add them to your HIIT workouts to amp up the fat-burning benefits.

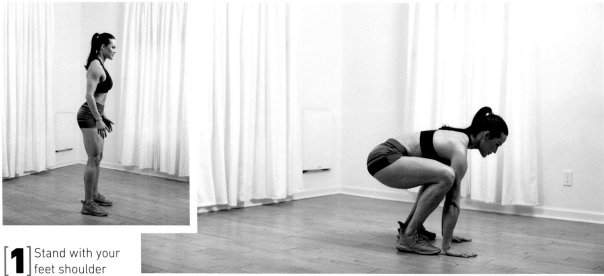

[1] Stand with your feet shoulder width apart and your hands at your sides.

[2] Quickly squat down, placing your hands on the floor.

[3] Kick your feet out behind you to come into a high plank position.

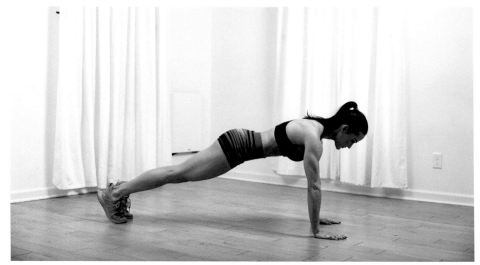

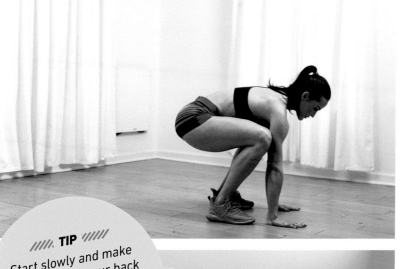

[4] Keeping your hands on the floor, jump your feet forward and back to your hands.

TIP

Start slowly and make sure you keep your back flat and wrists straight. Once you become more proficient, you can add more speed.

[5] Explosively jump straight up, extending your hands straight above your head, and then land back in the starting position.

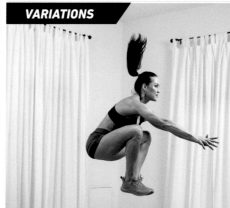

TUCK JUMP BURPEE (MORE CHALLENGING) Perform the exercise as instructed, but instead of jumping up from the burpee wth straight legs, jump up and tuck your knees to your chest.

BURPEE WITH DUMBBELLS (MORE CHALLENGING) Stand with dumbbells at your sides, and then get into a squat position, holding the dumbbells on the mat just in front of your feet. Balancing on the dumbbells, jump your feet back into a plank position. Perform a push up, and then jump your feet forward again into the squat position with your arms extended downward. As you begin to stand up, curl the dumbbells, keeping them close to your body, and then pressing them overhead.

TARGETS /// quads, hip flexors, glutes (primary); hamstrings, core (secondary)
EQUIPMENT /// none

HIGH KNEES

One of the most effective cardio moves you can do is a sprint. When most people picture sprints, they think about running on a track; however, with some modifications, you can sprint at home. Sprints not only train the entire body, they also can burn a tremendous number of calories, boost power, and actually help build muscle since they're an anaerobic exercise.

TRAIN THE RIGHT WAY

DO: Focus on the motion of driving your knees upward, rather than traveling forward.

DON'T: Tuck your chin or look down to check your form. (This will round your back and loosen your core.)

[**1**] Stand tall with your arms at your sides and your feet positioned a little less than shoulder width apart. Rise up onto your toes to prepare to sprint, and then lean forward slightly with your upper body.

[**2**] Quickly drive one knee upward so that your upper leg reaches parallel to the floor while simultaneously swinging your opposite arm forward. Swing your elbows through your hips and keep your upper body tall.

[**3**] Repeat the movement with the opposite arm and leg, alternating as you go and repeating the movement in a continuous motion so that you are running in place.

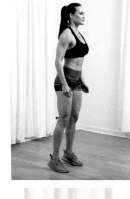

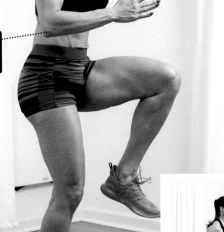

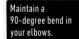

Maintain a 90-degree bend in your elbows.

VARIATIONS

BANDED HIGH KNEES (MORE CHALLENGING) Anchor a resistance band to a secure object at slightly lower than hip height. Step into the loop facing away from the anchor, and place the band around your hip bones. Walk forward to create tension in the band. Perform the exercise as instructed, leaning forward slightly more to push against the resistance of the band.

HIGH KNEES SKIPS Hop on one leg while driving the opposite knee toward your chest and opposite arm forward. Repeat on the opposite side.

TARGETS /// **delts, chest, core (primary); total body (secondary)**
EQUIPMENT /// **none**

SHADOW BOXING

A little creativity can go a long way when you're training at home. There's no treadmill or exercise bike when you're training at home, and that's a good thing! Shadow boxing works great as a warm-up, as an add-on between sets, or as a fat-burning exercise at the end of a workout. You can boost mindfulness, improve mind-muscle connection, and hit every muscle in the body with this exercise.

[**1**] Stand with one leg stepped back and your feet positioned shoulder width apart and turned diagonally. Stand with your body weight through the balls of your feet and with soft knees. Tuck your chin down slightly, lean forward slightly, and hold your fists just under your chin with your elbows tucked in.

[**2**] Begin bouncing slightly between your left and right feet. As your weight shifts to your front leg, simultaneously jab the air with the hand on the front leg side and then pull your arm back quickly.

[**3**] As your weight shifts to the back leg, punch with a cross and drive your back hip forward. Switch between jabs and crosses.

// TIP //
You can work on just jabs and then crosses or combine them quickly to work on speed and cardio.

VARIATIONS

SHADOW BOXING WITH LIGHT DUMBBELLS (MORE CHALLENGING)
Do the movement as instructed, but while holding light dumbbells.

TARGETS /// **total body**
EQUIPMENT /// **dumbbell**

DUMBBELL SWING

You may be familiar with kettlebell swings, but not every home-gym bodybuilder has access to kettlebells. No worries! This total body exercise can also be performed with a dumbbell. Add dumbbell swings to your warm-up, to burn calories between sets, or incorporate them into fat-burning circuits. You'll get leaner and more powerful, and you'll do it in less time.

TRAIN THE RIGHT WAY

DO: Keep your back flat and your head neutral as you perform the exercise.

DON'T: Use your arms to pull the dumbbell upward.

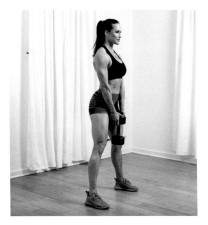

[**1**] Stand with your feet positioned just wider than shoulder width apart. Grasp the top of a dumbbell and wrap your fingers and thumbs around it. Hold the dumbbell in front of your body with your arms extended downward.

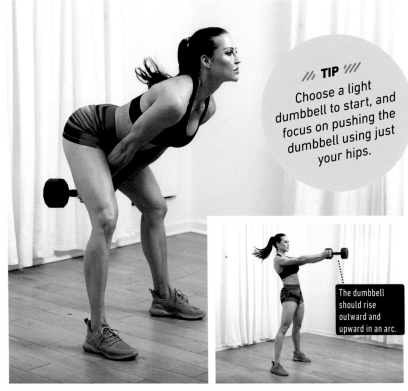

/// **TIP** ///
Choose a light dumbbell to start, and focus on pushing the dumbbell using just your hips.

The dumbbell should rise outward and upward in an arc.

VARIATIONS

DOUBLE-ARM DUMBBELL SWING Grasp two dumbbells and hold them at your sides. Squat down and use your hips to swing the dumbbells upward in an arc and outward. Squat down as the dumbbells return to your sides and repeat.

[**2**] Squat down slightly, keeping your arms extended, and then hinge at the hips as you swing the dumbbell back and between your legs.

[**3**] Use your hips to push the dumbbell forward until your arms reach parallel to the floor and your upper body stands tall, using your arms to guide the dumbbell. Bring the dumbbell back down between your legs as you squat down again.

TARGETS /// **quads, hip flexors, glutes (primary); hamstrings, core, calves (secondary)**

EQUIPMENT /// **none**

WALL SPRINT

This exercise enables you to perfect your sprint form without ever hitting the track or experiencing the wear and tear that's commonly associated with sprinting. You'll also boost your speed and power, and burn fat in the process. Using a wall helps you get into proper sprint form as you're able to lean forward into a powerful position, but without actually moving forward.

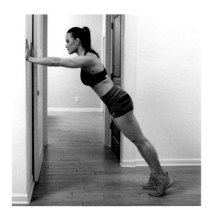

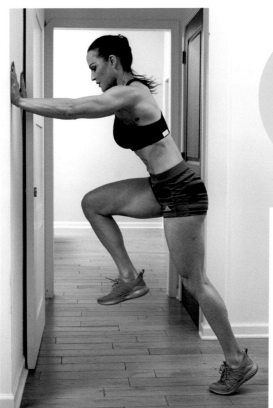

//// **TIP** ////
Keep your entire body tight, and actively push against the wall.

[1] Stand facing a wall with your feet positioned shoulder width apart. Extend your arms straight out in front of you, and place your palms flat on the wall. Step back until your body reaches about 45 degrees from the floor, shifting your body weight onto your toes.

[2] Drive one knee upward until the upper leg reaches parallel to the floor, making sure to keep your core tight and your foot dorsiflexed (toes angled up toward shin).

[3] Bring your leg back to the starting point and repeat on the other side. Repeat the sequence continuously.

VARIATIONS

HIGH KNEES WALL MARCH (EASIER) Get into the starting position as instructed. Perform the exercise slowly, squeezing the opposite hamstring and glute with each leg drive. (This variation is great for glute activation and perfecting form before moving on to wall sprints.)

WALL SIT Stand with your back to a wall and perform a squat, stepping forward until your back is pressed against the wall. Hold this isometric pose for the prescribed amount of time.

TARGETS /// **glutes, hamstrings, quads (primary); calves (secondary)**
EQUIPMENT /// **none**

POP SQUAT

Work on explosiveness, build strength and endurance, and hit every muscle in the legs and glutes with pop squats. This do-anywhere exercise is versatile—it can be used as part of a warm-up, in between sets to boost your heart rate, as a finisher, or as part of a cardio circuit. Keep the squats shallow, and push your weight through your toes to emphasize the quads. Squat deeper with weight through your heels to target the glutes more.

TRAIN THE RIGHT WAY

DO: Keep your upper body tall and your core tight.

DON'T: Allow your form to get sloppy as you get tired. Stay present and focused on performing the exercise properly.

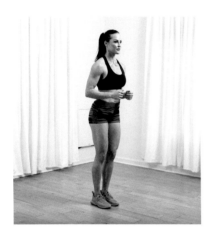

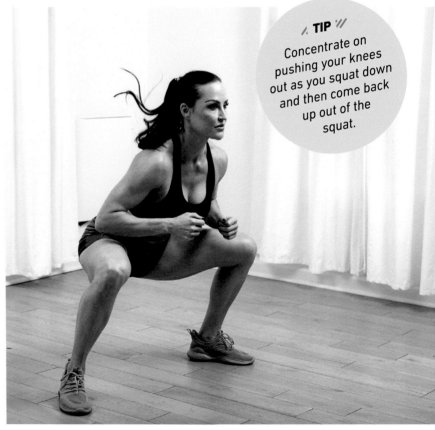

/. TIP '/
Concentrate on pushing your knees out as you squat down and then come back up out of the squat.

[1] Begin in a standing position with your hands out in front of you and your feet together.

[2] Quickly perform a small jump to drop into a squat, "pop" up out of the squat to jump back into the starting position. Repeat the sequence continuously.

VARIATIONS

WEIGHTED POP SQUAT (MORE CHALLENGING) Grasp a light dumbbell with a goblet hold. Perform the exercise as instructed.

SUMO SQUAT JACK Jump into a sumo squat position (a wide-legged squat with the toes pointing outward), and instead of popping back up into a standing position, perform a jumping jack. As your arms come down, jump back down into a sumo squat position.

JUMP SQUAT (MORE CHALLENGING) This is a more explosive plyometric variation. From a squat position, explode upward using your legs and arms. Land softly in a squat position and repeat. (Limit the reps to 10 or less.)

TARGETS /// quads, hamstrings, glutes (primary); calves (secondary)
EQUIPMENT /// bench

DYNAMIC STEP-UP

When training at home, targeting fast twitch muscles can be challenging. In a gym, fast twitch muscles are usually worked with very heavy weights and low reps. But since most home gyms aren't stocked with power racks, platforms, and stacks of weight plates, incorporating explosive movements is the best way to hit those fast twitch muscle fibers.

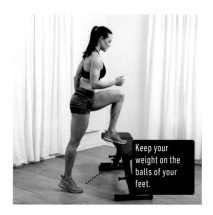

Keep your weight on the balls of your feet.

[1] Place one foot on the bench and one on the floor. Raise the arm that is opposite the raised leg upward while simultaneously pulling the opposite arm back.

TIP

To make the exercise more comfortable, try to keep your body weight centered between your front and rear legs.

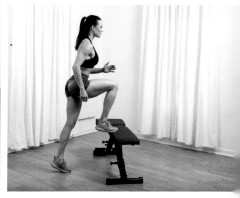

VARIATIONS

BEGINNER DYNAMIC STEP-UP (EASIER) Keep most of your body weight on the rear leg and stand tall. Jump and switch legs, making sure to swing the opposite arm with each jump.

WEIGHTED STEP-UP (MORE CHALLENGING) Hold dumbbells at your sides. Begin with both feet on the floor and quickly step up on the bench, driving the opposite knee upward until it reaches parallel to the floor. Step down and repeat on the opposite side.

[2] Jump up by pushing off of both feet and switching your legs mid-air. (As you switch legs, use your arms to counterbalance by swinging the opposite arm forward.)

[3] Land with your opposite foot on the bench and your opposite arm forward. Repeat in a continuous motion, switching the arm and leg positions with each jump.

TARGETS /// chest, triceps (primary); abs, shoulders (secondary)
EQUIPMENT /// yoga mat

PLYO PUSH-UP

Overall power and strength is increased when you're able to incorporate upper-body plyometrics into your training. This can directly enhance your lifts in the gym as you'll be able to press more. It can also improve life outside of the gym as your balance and body awareness will be better.

TRAIN THE RIGHT WAY

DO: Maintain a plank position throughout the exercise.

DON'T: Crank your neck upward or allow your hips to sag.

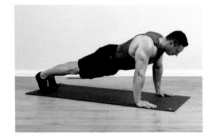

[1] Rise into a high plank position with your hands positioned a bit wider than shoulder width apart.

[2] Lower down into a push-up with your body close to the floor.

[3] Explosively push your body upward, trying to make your hands leave the floor. Land as softly as possible, reset, and repeat.

VARIATIONS

PLYO PUSH-UP ON KNEES (EASIER) Rather than in a full plank position, perform the exercise on your knees with your feet crossed.

SHOULDER TAP PUSH-UP (MORE CHALLENGING) Perform a push-up, and while in the high plank position, touch one hand to the opposite shoulder. Repeat on the opposite side.

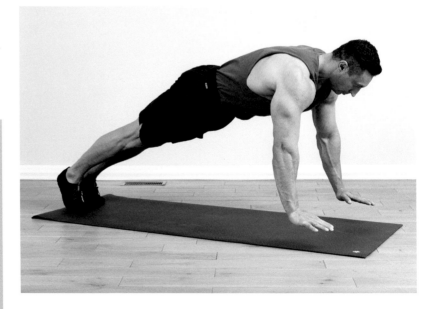

Pull your elbows back toward your ribcage.

TARGETS /// **core, shoulders, legs (primary); back, arms (secondary)**
EQUIPMENT /// **none**

BEAR CRAWL

Improve agility, strengthen your core, burn calories, and increase coordination with bear crawls. Often seen in obstacle courses and boot camps, this exercise will hit almost every muscle in your body. You can add it to conditioning circuits or use it as a workout finisher or even part of your warm-up to quickly elevate your heart rate. Though you won't need any equipment, having an open or long and narrow space, like a hallway, to perform it in can make it easier.

TRAIN THE RIGHT WAY

DO: Keep your back flat as you crawl.

DON'T: Allow your knees to touch the floor.

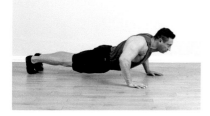

[1] Drop into a push-up position. Bend your arms to lower your upper body closer to the floor.

[2] Move forward by simultaneously moving one arm and the opposite leg forward.

[3] Advance the opposite arm and leg forward, alternating the movement on each side to continuously crawl forward.

VARIATIONS

BACKWARD BEAR CRAWL Perform the exercise in reverse, moving backward as you go. This variation can be added to the bear crawl to eliminate the need to turn around.

BEAR CRAWL WITH DUMBBELLS (MORE CHALLENGING) Grasp light dumbbells and perform the exercise as instructed. (Take extra care if your dumbbells are round and you're training on a hard surface.)

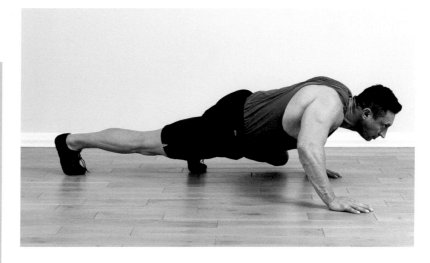

Keep your core tight.

Make sure your knees don't touch the floor.

TARGETS /// **quads, core, calves (primary);**
hamstrings, glutes, upper body (secondary)
EQUIPMENT /// **bench**

INCLINE MOUNTAIN CLIMBER

The incline mountain climber puts you into "drive phase" or the acceleration position of a sprint, which can improve speed, explosiveness, and power. You'll be able to elevate your heart rate quickly and train your entire body. It's also a sneaky way to strengthen your core, as you'll be in a high plank position the entire time and must use your core to stabilize your body.

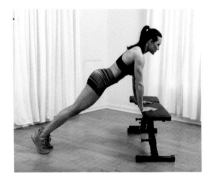

[1] Place both hands on a bench with your arms spaced shoulder width apart and perpendicular to the floor. Get into a high plank position with a neutral spine.

[2] In a continuous motion, quickly drive one knee up to your chest, snap it back to the starting position, and repeat on the opposite side. Repeat the movement in a continuous back-and-forth fashion as if you're running in place.

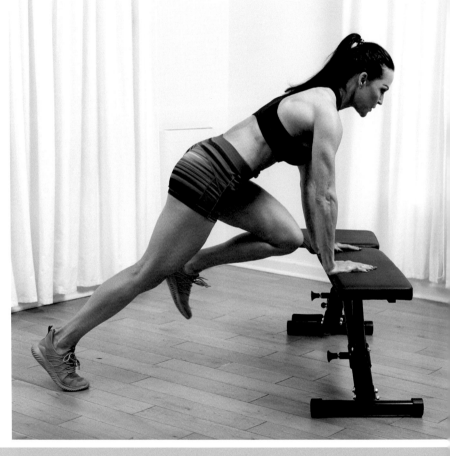

VARIATIONS

MOUNTAIN CLIMBER Perform the exercise as instructed, but with your hands placed flat on the floor.

SLOW-MOTION MOUNTAIN CLIMBER Get into a high plank position and slowly drive one knee to the elbow on the same side of your body. As you drive your knee, crunch your abs and emphasize the contraction. Repeat on the opposite side.

TARGETS /// **quads, glutes, hamstrings (primary);**
abs, arms, upper back (secondary)
EQUIPMENT /// **dumbbells**

DUMBBELL THRUSTER

This advanced multi-joint exercise hits most of the major muscles in the body. It's basically a seamless combination of a squat and then a shoulder press. Master this move and your form on most basic lifts will improve, as will your strength. Dumbbell thrusters can be used as a warm-up, or they can be added to your HIIT or cardio circuits for a fat-burning boost. Since this is an advanced move, pay close attention to form when starting, and only use light dumbbells.

TRAIN THE RIGHT WAY

DO: Keep your chest up as you squat, and push your weight through your heels.

DON'T: Allow your elbows to drop as this can cause your chest to drop and your lower back to round.

[1] Grasp two dumbbells using a neutral grip, and hold them close to your shoulders, with your elbows directly underneath the dumbbells and your upper arms just below parallel to the floor. Place your feet shoulder width apart or a bit wider.

[2] Keeping your chest tall, squat to parallel while keeping the dumbbells in place.

[3] Pushing your weight through your heels and keeping your chest tall and your core tight, push your body back up to the standing position, as you begin to reach standing, press the dumbbells upward as you would in a neutral-grip shoulder press until your arms are fully extended overhead. Lower the dumbbells back down to the starting position and repeat.

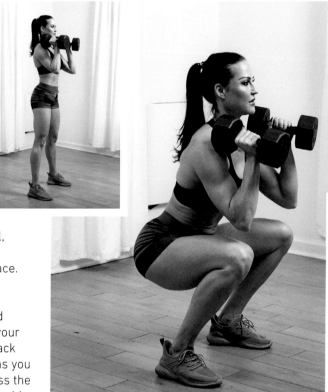

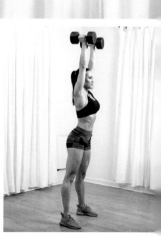

VARIATIONS

SINGLE-ARM THRUSTERS Perform the exercise using just one dumbbell at a time. (This improves core strength.)

ROTATIONAL THRUSTERS Instead of standing up straight, rotate your body to one side and pivot the opposite foot to allow for rotation. As you lower the dumbbells back down, rotate back to square and then repeat the movement on the opposite side.

INDEX

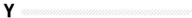